Leukemia Next Level

With Orthodox and Alternative Treatment

Preface

I have written this book so that the patients suffering from Leukemia can understand the disease in detail and choose a suitable treatment for them. This book provides simple approach about the clinical symptoms, complications, diagnosis, staging and treatments. In the last 15 years there has been considerable research and progress in the field of clinical studies, etiology, pathology, diagnosis and treatment of Leukemia.

In this book, I have written in detail about Orthodox and Alternative Treatment. I have also included Budwig Protocol, which is the best alternative treatment and gives authentic success. Patient can carefully select the right treatment for him. This book has up to date information.

Dr. O.P.Verma

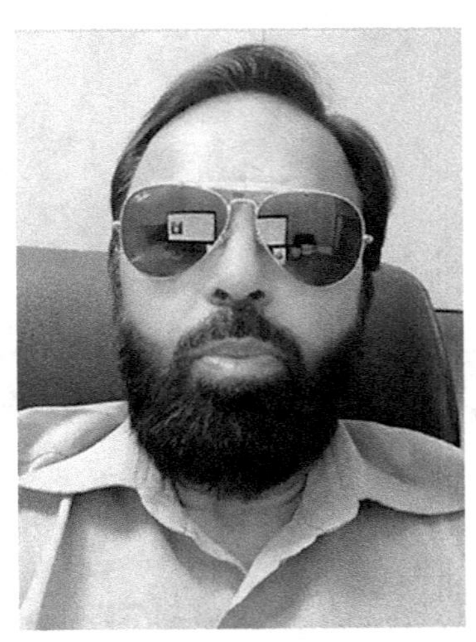

Written by
Dr. O.P.Verma
M.B.B.S., M.R.S.H. (London)
Budwig Wellness
7-B-43, Mahaveer Nagar III, Kota (Raj.)
https://gobudwig.com
+919460816360

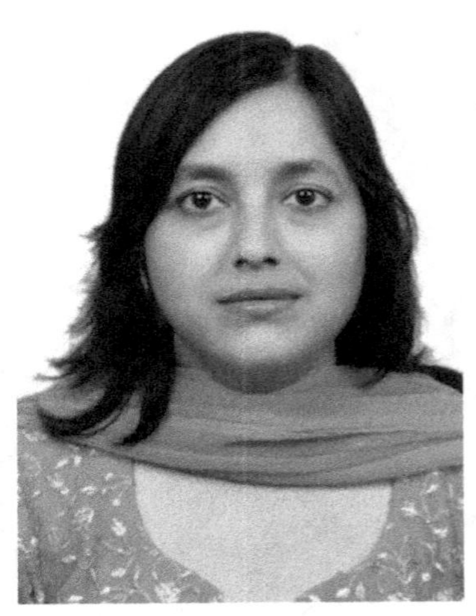

Edited by
Aishvarya Sharma
Senior Manager
Software A.G.
Bengaluru, Karnataka
B.Tech., I.I.T. B.H.U., Varanasi U.P.

Table of Content

Leukemia

Leukemia is a group of blood-related cancers that affect white blood cell replication in the bone marrow. The abnormal cells crowd out the healthy cells, which affects their ability to fight infection and impedes the production of blood cells.

There are four major types of the disease. □ Most of the time, its cause is unknown, but risk factors include genetics, smoking, radiation, and environmental exposures.

Symptoms are non-specific and may include anemia, frequent infections, bruising, and weight loss.

Leukemia may be suspected on blood tests, but further testing is needed to make the diagnosis. Treatment□depends on the type and may include chemotherapy, a stem cell transplant, and/or other options.

While acute leukemia is the most common cancer in childhood, in general, leukemia is more common in older adults.

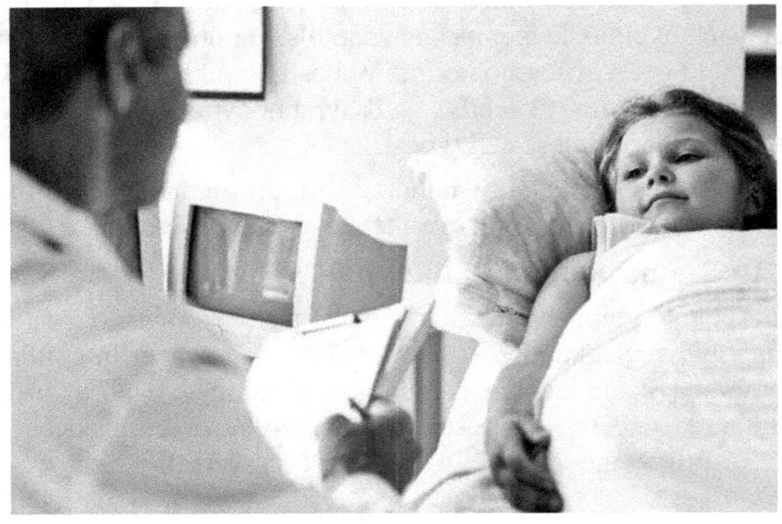

Types of Leukemia

Leukemia is first classified as acute or chronic and as either myelogenous or lymphocytic.

Acute leukemia arises from immature cells in the bone marrow (myeloblasts or lymphoblasts). These cells do not function like fully mature ones in fighting off infections. In addition, they often crowd the bone marrow, preventing the production of other blood cells such as red blood cells, other white blood cells, and platelets. Without treatment, acute leukemia often progress very rapidly.

Chronic leukemia arises from mature, but abnormal white blood cells. These cancers grow much more slowly and may be discovered accidentally when a blood count is done for another reason.

Myelogenous vs. Lymphocytic

All of the blood cells derive from pluripotential stem cells in the bone marrow thanks to a process called hematopoiesis. These cells differentiate into either myeloid cells (the myeloid cell line) or lymph cells (the lymphoid cell line). Myeloid cells differentiate into red blood cells, platelets, and the type of cells found in myeloid leukemia: neutrophils, monocytes, and more. Lymphoid cells differentiate into either B lymphocytes (B cells) or T lymphocytes (T cells), and lymphocytic leukemias may begin in either of these cell types.

Leukemia is actually hundreds of different diseases on a molecular level, with no two leukemias being exactly alike.

Acute Lymphocytic Leukemia (ALL)

Acute lymphocytic leukemia, also known as acute lymphoblastic leukemia, is the most common cancer in children. (Combined, acute leukemias are responsible for around a third of childhood cancers.) That said, around 40% of cases occur in adults. While the disease was almost universally fatal a few decades ago, it is now curable in the majority of children diagnosed.

Chronic Lymphocytic Leukemia (CLL)

Chronic lymphocytic leukemia is the most common leukemia in adults and is often diagnosed before any symptoms develop. In some ways, it is very similar to some lymphomas and is treated in a similar fashion.

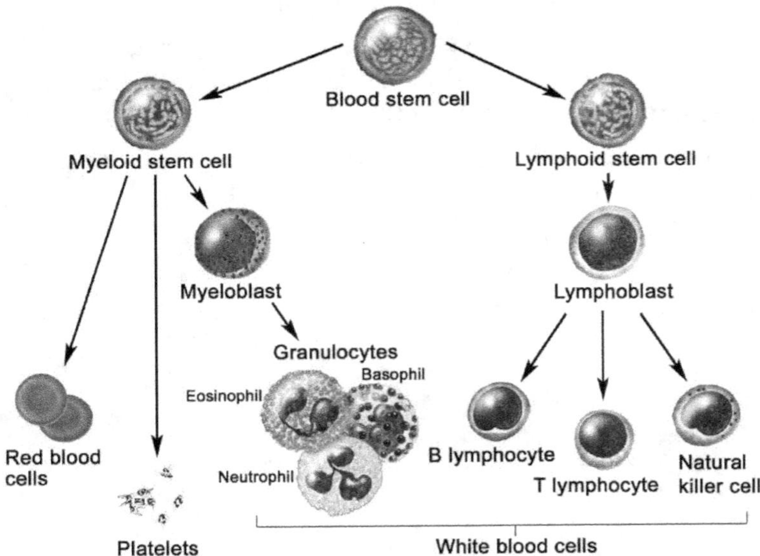

Acute Myeloid Leukemia (AML)

Although often thought of as childhood cancer, acute myeloid leukemia (acute myelogenous leukemia) is actually more common in adults. In fact, it is the most common form of acute leukemia in these individuals.

The treatment is more aggressive than for other forms of leukemia and often requires in-hospital treatment for the first few weeks. There are several different subtypes of acute myeloid leukemia that differ in many ways, including the prognosis.

One type of AML, acute promyelocytic leukemia, is treated with additional medications specific to the disease. It has the best prognosis of these cancers.

Chronic Myeloid Leukemia (CML)

Chronic myeloid leukemia (CML) is much more common in older adults. CML was the first type of cancer to be successfully controlled with targeted therapies—drugs that zero in on specific abnormalities in the growth of the cells.

These treatments have changed the prognosis from almost universally fatal (eventually) to largely controllable over the long-term with continued treatment.

Both CML and CLL have the potential to become acute leukemia over time.

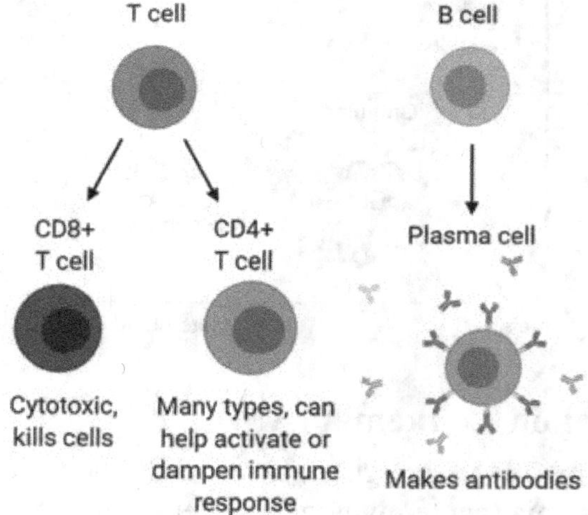

Difference between Leukemia and Lymphoma

Both leukemias and lymphomas are considered "blood-related cancers" or "liquid cancers," but there are differences. While there are exceptions, some major differences between leukemias and lymphomas include:

Location of origin: Leukemias begin in the bone marrow, whereas lymphomas begin in lymph nodes.

Symptoms: Lymphomas commonly present with enlarged lymph nodes or constitutional symptoms such as weight loss, night sweats, and fever. Leukemia often presents due to signs of low levels of the blood cells made in the bone marrow, such as pallor, lightheadedness, and fatigue (due to a low red blood cell count), infections (due to improperly functioning white blood cells), and bruising and bleeding (due to a low platelet count).

Incidence: Lymphomas are more common than leukemias.

Age of onset: Some types of leukemias are more common in children, whereas lymphomas are, by and large, more common in adults.

Causes and Risk Factors of Leukemia

Leukemia is due to a series of mutations in genes that control the growth of cells, which leads to their uncontrolled growth in the bone marrow. While the exact causes of this are unknown, several risk factors for the disease have been identified. Known risk factors vary with the different types of leukemia but include radiation (from atomic bomb exposures to medical radiation), exposures to chemicals such as benzene and pesticides, previous chemotherapy, some infections, and certain genetic conditions. There are others still under investigation as well, such as radon.

Chronic leukemia is much more common in older adults, and though acute leukemia is often thought of as being a childhood cancer, acute myeloid leukemia is actually much more common in adults. For

Confirmed and Probable Risk Factors

There are several risk factors for the development of leukemia that have been documented in a number of studies. A risk factor is something that is associated with an increased risk of developing leukemia but does not necessarily cause the disease. Some of these include:

Age

Age as a risk factor for leukemia varies widely with the type of leukemia. Together, acute lymphocytic leukemia (ALL) and acute myelogenous leukemia (AML) account for 30% of childhood cancers.

While many people consider these diseases pediatric cancers, AML is actually much more common in adults (the average age at diagnosis is 68).

Around 40 percent of cases of ALL are in adults; when diagnosed in childhood, it is most common in children under the age of 5 years.

Chronic lymphocytic leukemia (CLL) and chronic myelogenous leukemia (CML) are much more common in older adults and are very uncommon in people under the age of 40.

Gender

The primary types of leukemia (AML, ALL, CML, and CLL) are slightly more common in males than females, but the reason for this is unknown.

Birth Weight

Children who have high birth weights (weight at birth greater than 8.9 pounds or 4000 grams) have a greater risk of developing ALL.

Ethnicity

Racial differences in incidence differ between the types of leukemia. ALL has the highest incidence in Hispanic whites, followed by non-Hispanic whites and Asian and Pacific Islanders, with the lowest incidence in blacks.

CLL is more common in non-Hispanic whites, followed by blacks, with the lowest incidence in Hispanics and Asian and Pacific Islanders.

AML is similar among people of different ethnic backgrounds during childhood, but in adults is more common in non-Hispanic whites.

CML is most common in non-Hispanic whites followed by blacks and then Hispanics, with the lowest incidence in Asian and Pacific Islanders.

Radiation

Some types of radiation are known risk factors for leukemia, and others are only possible risk factors. There are two primary types of radiation:

Non-ionizing radiation: This type of radiation is fairly weak and includes the type that is emitted from a cell phone or computer terminal. While some concerns have been raised, such as the concern about brain tumor risk and cell phones, the risk is considered relatively small.

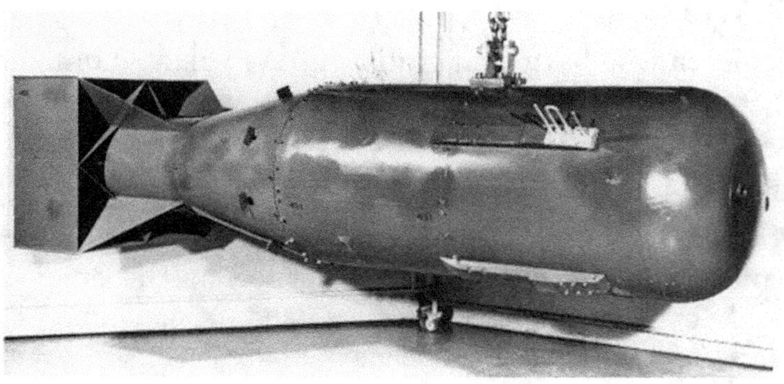

Ionizing radiation: In contrast, ionizing radiation has been linked to leukemia. This type of radiation has much more energy—enough to break certain chemical bonds, remove electrons from atoms, and damage DNA in cells.

There are a number of different ways in which ionizing radiation has been associated with leukemia. These include:

- **Atomic bomb radiation:** Survivors of the Hiroshima and Nagasaki atomic bombings had a significantly increased risk of developing leukemia.

- **Nuclear accidents:** Survivors of the 1986 Chernobyl nuclear reactor disaster had an increased risk of leukemia two to five years after the meltdown. Those who were highly exposed had twice the risk of developing leukemia as those not exposed.

- **Medical diagnostic radiation:** Ionizing radiation was found to be carcinogenic (or cancer-causing) only a few years after X-rays were discovered, and concern has been raised in recent years over the danger of too much medical radiation, particularly in children. The risk varies, with imaging tests such as CT scans, bone scans, and PET scans involving much more radiation than plain X-rays. (MRI scans use magnets and do not involve exposure to radiation.)

- **Medical therapeutic radiation:** Radiation therapy for cancer can increase the risk of developing leukemia (especially AML), with the risk highest in the period five to nine years after radiation. The risk varies with the site of radiation as well as the dose used.

- **Radioactive iodine therapy:** Receiving radioactive iodine therapy as a treatment for hyperthyroidism or thyroid cancer is associated with an increased risk of leukemia, with the risk of AML being 80% higher than for those who didn't receive this therapy.□ The risk is even higher for CML, with those exposed having a risk 3.5 times higher than average.

- **Air and space travel:** Air flight, especially over the far north, involves exposure to cosmic radiation, but this amount of ionizing radiation is relatively small. The leukemia risk from space travel due to galactic cosmic rays, however, is a subject of great interest among those looking at travel to places such as Mars in the future.

- **Radioactive materials:** Uranium mining as an occupation increases the risk of leukemia. There has also been concern about exposure to radioactive material in tobacco products, which pick up these materials in the soil where they are grown.

Previous Chemotherapy

While the benefits of chemotherapy usually far outweigh the risks, some chemotherapy drugs can predispose a person to leukemia later on. This is true even for the drugs commonly used for early-stage breast cancer.

For most of these drugs, the risk begins to increase two years after treatment and peaks between five and 10 years after treatment.

AML is the form of leukemia most often associated with chemotherapy, but ALL has also been linked to the treatment.[20] Examples of drugs associated with leukemia include Cytoxan (cyclophosphamide); Leukeran (chlorambucil); VePesid (etoposide); Vumon (teniposide); Gleostine, CeeNu, and CCNSB (lomustine); Gliadel and BiCNU (carmustine); Myleran (busulfan); Mustargen (mechlorethamine); and Novantrone (mitoxantrone).

Drugs such as Adriamycin (doxorubicin) and other anthracyclines, Platinol (cisplatin) and other platinum drugs, and bleomycin have been associated with leukemia but less commonly than the drugs mentioned earlier.

Medical Conditions

Some medical conditions are associated with an elevated risk of developing leukemia. Myelodysplastic syndromes are disorders of the bone marrow that have been referred to as "preleukemia" and carry a significant risk of developing into AML (up to 30%). Other conditions such as essential thrombocytopenia, primary myelofibrosis, and polycythemia vera also carry an increased risk.

Furthermore, people who are immunosuppressed, such as those who take immunosuppressive medications due to an organ transplant, have a significantly increased risk of developing leukemia.

Associations have been noted between leukemia in adults and medical conditions such as inflammatory bowel disease (ulcerative colitis and Crohn's disease), rheumatoid arthritis, systemic lupus erythematosus (lupus), celiac disease, and pernicious anemia, among others. However, a large 2012 study looking into these associations only found an increased risk relationship with ulcerative colitis and AML, and peptic ulcer disease and CML.

Genetic syndromes may also increase the risk of leukemia.

Smoking

Adding to the list of cancers caused by smoking, tobacco use is associated with a significantly increased risk of AML.

At the current time, it's thought that around 20 percent of AML cases are linked to smoking.

There is some evidence that leukemia in children may be linked with parent's smoking, and mothers exposed to secondhand smoke appear to have a slightly elevated risk of developing ALL.

Home and Occupational Exposures

There are a number of exposures that have been associated with leukemia, though the risk varies with the different types of the disease. Some of the substances have been linked clearly in many studies, while others are still uncertain. Some exposures of interest include:

- **Benzene:** Benzene is a known carcinogen that is present in a number of materials, such as some paints, solvents, plastics, pesticides, detergents, and unleaded gasoline. Benzene is also a byproduct of the combustion of coal. Benzene in tobacco smoke is thought to be one of the reasons why smoking is strongly linked to AML. Maternal and childhood exposure to paint at home is associated with an elevated risk of ALL. Home use of petroleum solvents is associated with an increased risk of childhood AML.

- **Home pesticide exposures:** Pesticide exposure during pregnancy and childhood appears to be associated with an increased risk of leukemia, according to several studies.

- **Contaminated drinking water:** An increased risk of leukemia was found among those at a U.S. Marine Corp base camp in North Carolina that was contaminated by a solvent between 1950 and 1985.

- **Formaldehyde:** Medical workers and embalmers have an increased risk of myeloid leukemias. While exposure is common in these workers, but many people are exposed to formaldehyde through the "off-gassing" of formaldehyde from pressed wood products (such as particleboard, plywood, and fiberboard). Formaldehyde exposure such as this is considered to be a known carcinogen, but it's not clear what level of exposure (amount or duration) might be a problem. Other sources of formaldehyde include some glues and adhesives, some insulation materials, and some paper product coatings. Like benzene, formaldehyde is also found in tobacco smoke.

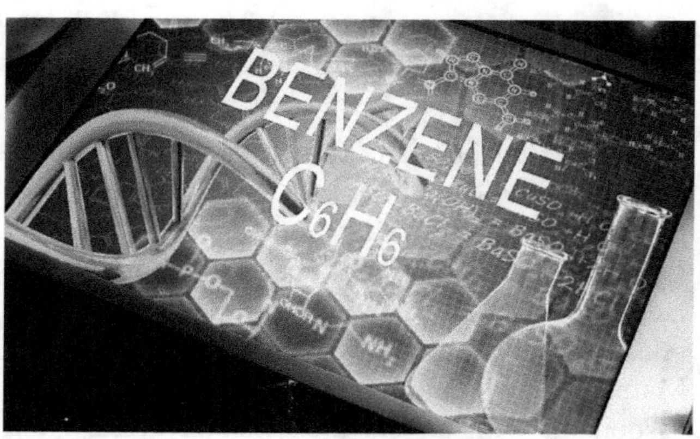

Noting that the incidence of childhood leukemia has been increasing in California, studies looking at environmental exposures that may be associated with this risk are in progress.

Infections

Infection with the human T-cell leukemia virus (HTLV-1) increases the risk of leukemia. The virus is a retrovirus (similar to HIV) and infects the type of white blood cells known as T lymphocytes or T cells. HTLV-1 is spread in a way similar to HIV; it can be transmitted through blood transfusions, through sexual contact, by sharing needles among IV drug abusers, and from a mother to a child during delivery or through breastfeeding.

HTLV-1 is relatively uncommon in the United States, but is found in the Caribbean (especially Haiti and Jamaica), Japan, central and west Africa, and Middle East (especially Iran). It's thought that between 1 and 4% of people who are exposed to the virus will develop leukemia; the most common age of onset is between 30 and 50.

Alcohol

While alcohol consumption is linked with a number of cancers, a 2014 study□ found no association between alcohol use and the four major types of leukemia. There has been a link noted, however, between maternal alcohol consumption during pregnancy and AML in children born to these mothers.

Possible Risk Factors

In addition to known and probable risk factors for leukemia, there are several risk factors that are being evaluated for their association with leukemia. Some possible risk factors include:

Western Diet

With many types of leukemia, especially acute leukemia in children, there appears to be little association with dietary practices. In CLL, however, the most common type of leukemia in American adults, diet may play a role.

A 2018 study in Spain found that those who ate a Western diet were 63 percent more likely to develop CLL than those who consumed a Prudent diet or Mediterranean diet.

Sucralose

There has been controversy surrounding a possible connection between the artificial sweetener sucralose and cancer.

Sucralose (with brand names including Sugar free and others) was approved in 1999 and is currently in thousands of products worldwide.

Despite a multitude of reassuring studies prior to its approval, a 2016 Italian study on mice found that rodents who were exposed to sucralose throughout their lives (beginning in utero) had a significantly increased risk of developing leukemia.

It's important to note that this was an animal study, and the doses given were equivalent to an adult consuming four times the average amount of sucralose every single day. That said, with the popularity of sucralose as a sugar substitute, it's thought that young children could easily exceed the FDA's acceptable daily intake of 5 mg/kg daily.

(Keep in mind that, despite a focused concern about sucralose, questions have been raised about the use of other artificial sweeteners as well. Ideally, any of these products should be used sparingly in a healthy diet.)

Electromagnetic Fields (Power Lines)

Since 1979, when a study found an increased risk of leukemia in children who lived near high voltage power lines, a number of studies have looked at this possible association with mixed results. Some showed an increased risk with high levels of exposure, and others showed little, if any, effect. Three analyses that have compared results of studies to date (totaling 31 studies in all) found that high exposures (0.3 uT or higher) were associated with a 1.4 to 2.0 times increased risk of leukemia. This level of exposure, however, is not common. In these studies, only 0.5 to 3.0% of children had an exposure equal to or exceeding 0.3 uT.

Radon

At the current time, there is a possibility that radon in homes, a form of ionizing radiation, may increase the risk of chronic lymphocytic leukemia (CLL).

Radon is a well-known carcinogen, and it's thought that roughly 27,000 people die from radon-induced lung cancer each year in the United States.

Radon is an odorless, colorless gas, that is produced by the normal breakdown of uranium found in the soil and rocks beneath homes. Elevated levels have been found in all 50 states, and the only way to know if you are at risk is to do radon testing.

A 2016 study found that the areas in the United States where CLL is most common are also the regions known to have the highest radon levels (northern and central states). While the association between radon and leukemia is uncertain, some researchers propose that radon could lead to leukemia in a way similar to how it increases lung cancer risk.

Coffee and Tea

Coffee and tea have both been looked at with regard to the risk of leukemia, and the studies have been mixed. Some indicated an increased risk with more consumption, while others instead showed a potential protective effect (a reduced risk of leukemia). Since people metabolize coffee and tea in different ways (fast metabolizers vs. slow metabolizers), it could be that the effects vary between different people.

Sedentary Lifestyle

While some studies have found no association between level of physical activity and leukemia, a 2016 study found that people who engaged in more "leisure physical activity" were around

20% less likely to develop myeloid leukemias than those who were less active.

Genetics

The role of family history and genetics varies between the different types of leukemia.

ALL does not appear to run in families, with the exception being identical twins, in which one of the siblings in the pair has an increased risk of developing ALL if the other developed the disease before one year of age. That said, there are certain genetic syndromes that are associated with an increased risk of this type of leukemia.

In contrast, family history plays an important role in CLL.

People who have a first-degree family member who has had CLL (parent, sibling, or child) have more than twice the risk of developing the disease themselves.

A family history of AML in first-degree relatives increases risk, but the age at diagnosis is important. Siblings of children with AML have up to a four times higher risk of developing the disease, with the risk in identical twins being around 20%. In contrast, children who have a parent who has adult-onset leukemia do not appear to be at a higher risk.

Family history doesn't appear to play a significant role in the development of CML.

Genetic conditions☐ and syndromes that are associated with an increased risk of some types of leukemia include:

- Down syndrome (trisomy 21): People with Down syndrome have roughly a 20 % increased risk of developing leukemia (AML and ALL). The incidence is highest in children under the age of 5 years.
- Klinefelter's syndrome (XXY)
- Fanconi anemia☐
- Li-Fraumeni syndrome ☐

- Neurofibromatosis ☐
- Ataxia telangiectasia ☐
- Bloom syndrome
- Wiskott Aldrich syndrome
- Schwachman-Diamond syndrome
- Blackfan-Diamond syndrome
- Kostmann syndrome

Symptoms of Leukemia

The symptoms of leukemia may be very subtle at first and include fatigue, unexplained fever, abnormal bruising, headaches, excessive bleeding (such as frequent nosebleeds), unintentional weight loss, and frequent infections, to name a few. These, however, can be due to a wide range of causes. If related to leukemia, symptoms may hint at the type of the disease that is present, but many symptoms overlap and are not this specific. Leukemia cannot be diagnosed based on symptoms alone, but an awareness of them can suggest when further evaluation is needed.

Frequent Symptoms

The symptoms of leukemia in adults and children are similar. The most common symptoms are:

- Fatigue
- Frequent infections
- Enlarged lymph nodes
- Unexplained fevers
- Night sweats
- Bruising and excess bleeding
- Abdominal pain
- Bone and joint pain
- Headaches and other neurological symptoms
- Unintentional weight loss

Because many of these symptoms are vague and non-specific, people tend to explain them away, saying that they feel like they are catching a cold or they've been feeling run-down lately.

Symptoms of leukemia can be difficult to detect in younger children who may only able to communicate by crying. The only other signs may be as a lack of appetite, the refusal to eat, or the appearance of a limp due to a bone or joint pain.

Some of the symptoms are easier to understand in the context of the effect leukemia has on specific blood cells produced by the bone marrow, since many of the signs are related to either an excess or deficiency of these cells.

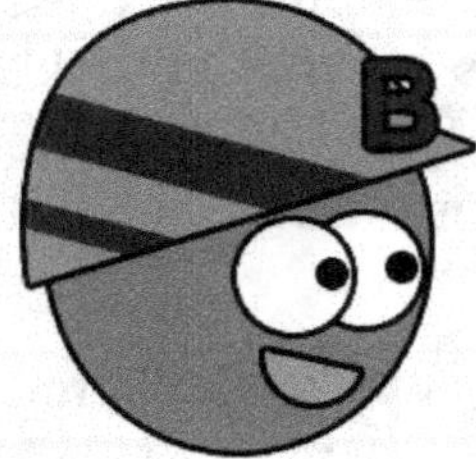
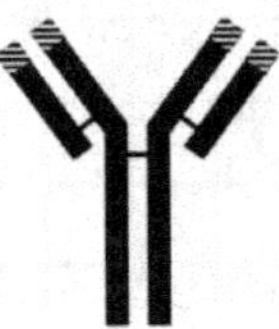

Leukemia affects white blood cells, but also frequently affects other cells produced by the bone marrow by interfering with their production or crowding out the bone marrow. Cells manufactured by the bone marrow include:

- **Red blood cells (RBCs):** Red blood cells carry oxygen to the tissues of the body. A low red blood cell count is referred to as anemia.

- **White blood cells (WBCs):** White blood cells are responsible for fighting off infections due to organisms such as bacteria and viruses. A low white blood cell count is referred to as leukopenia. One type of white blood cell, neutrophils, are particularly important in fighting off the bacteria that cause infections such as pneumonia. A deficiency of neutrophils is referred to as neutropenia.
- **Platelets:** Platelets or thrombocytes are the cells produced by the bone marrow that are responsible for blood clotting. A low platelet count is referred to as thrombocytopenia.

Fatigue

Excessive tiredness is a very common symptom of leukemia. Though there are many causes of fatigue, cancer fatigue tends to be more dramatic than the ordinary tiredness people feel when they lack sleep. The kind of fatigue associated with cancer often doesn't improve with a good night of rest and interferes with normal daily activities.

Cancer can cause fatigue in different ways. Leukemia-associated anemia depletes cells and tissues of oxygen, causing shortness of breath and weakness. Cancer can also decrease the production of serotonin and tryptophan key to physical and mental function.

Frequent Infections

Even when present in normal or increased numbers, cancerous white blood cells (leukemia) may not be able to adequately help your body fight off infection. In addition, the leukemia cells can crowd out other types of white blood cells in the bone marrow, preventing the body from ensuring an adequate supply.

As a result, people affected by leukemia are often very prone to developing infections. Common sites of infection include the mouth and throat, skin, lungs, urinary tract or bladder, and the area around the anus.

Enlarged Lymph Nodes

Sometimes, leukemia cells can accumulate in the lymph nodes and cause them to become swollen and tender. People may be able to feel abnormally enlarged lymph nodes (lymphadenopathy) in the neck (axillary lymph nodes), armpit (cervical lymph nodes), or groin, but lymph nodes that can't be directly palpated can also cause symptoms as well.

For example, enlarged lymph nodes in the chest (such as mediastinal lymph nodes) cannot be felt but may lead to shortness of breath, wheezing, or a cough.

Bruising or Excess Bleeding

When leukemia cells crowd the bone marrow, it can result in a decreased production of platelets, known as thrombocytopenia. Platelets are actually fragments of cells that clump together to slow or stop bleeding when an injury occurs to a blood vessel.

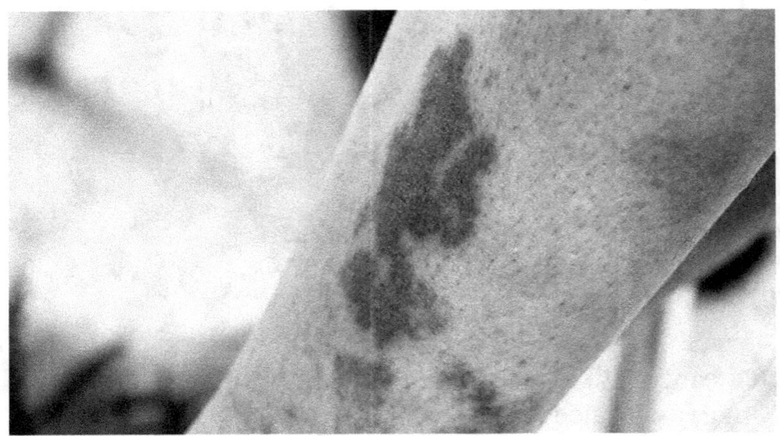

Leukemia-associated thrombocytopenia can take many forms, including easy bruising, skin spots (petechiae or purpura), heavy periods, nosebleeds, bleeding gums, hematuria (blood in urine), and hematochezia (blood in stools).

Unexplained Fevers

Fevers without an obvious source, such as infection, can be a symptom of any cancer, but especially blood-related cancers such as leukemia. A fever of unknown origin is defined as a fever of greater than 101 degrees that occurs frequently or lasts for more than three weeks with no obvious explanation.

Fevers associated with leukemia can have a number of possible causes, including underlying infections. In some cases, leukemia cells themselves can cause the body to release chemicals that stimulate the brain to raise body temperature.

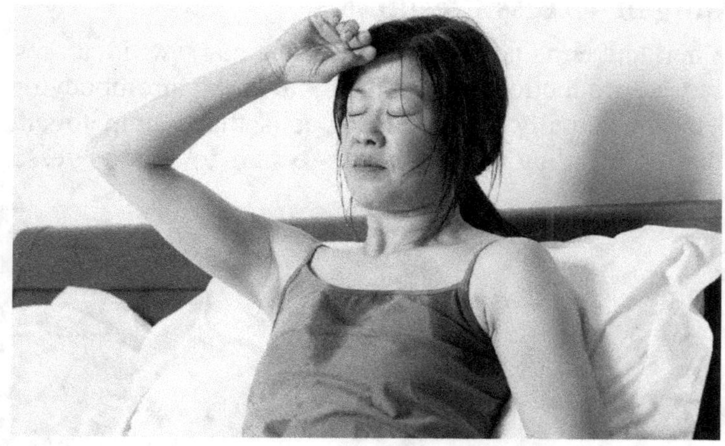

Night Sweats

Night sweats can be a symptom of cancer, especially blood-related cancers like leukemia. Unlike the common hot flashes or sweating associated with menopause, night sweats related to leukemia are often dramatic.

Night sweats are typically described as "drenching," soaking through clothing and bedding to the mattress below. While they are common at night, night sweats can also occur during the day and are never considered normal.

Abdominal Pain

Abnormal white blood cells may collect in the liver and spleen, causing your abdomen to swell and become uncomfortable. This type of swelling can also decrease your appetite or make you feel full early in a meal. Involvement of the spleen often causes pain in the right upper abdomen, whereas liver involvement often causes pain in the left upper abdomen.

Bone and Joint Pain

Bone and joint pain are most common in areas where there is a large amount of bone marrow, such as the pelvis (hips) or breastbone (sternum). This is caused by the crowding of the marrow with excessive numbers of abnormal white blood cells. In children, parents may notice that a child is limping or not walking normally without any form of injury to explain the symptom.

Headaches and Other Neurological Symptoms

Headaches and other neurologic symptoms such as seizures, dizziness, visual changes, nausea, and vomiting may occur when leukemia cells invade the fluid surrounding the brain and spinal cord (cerebrospinal fluid).

Unintentional Weight Loss

Unexplained weight loss is a classic sign of all cancers and is generally suggestive of a more advanced malignancy. In some cases, persistent fatigue and unintended weight loss are the symptoms that compel some people to seek a diagnosis.

Unexplained weight loss is defined as the loss of 5 percent or more of your body weight over a span of six to 12 months. The symptom is more common with chronic leukemias than acute leukemias.

By Type

While the symptoms above may be found with nearly any type of leukemia, there are some symptoms that are more common with different types of the disease.

Acute leukemias are characterized by immature white blood cells that do not function properly, leading to a more visible array of symptoms. With chronic leukemias, the cells may function to some degree and, as such, may have less obvious symptoms.

Symptoms related to the different subtypes of leukemia include:

Acute Lymphocytic Leukemia (ALL)

The symptoms of acute lymphocytic leukemia often develop rapidly over the course of days or a few weeks. If ALL spreads to the central nervous system, symptoms such as headaches, blurry vision, dizziness, and sometimes seizures may occur. When ALL spreads to the chest, shortness of breath and a cough may occur.

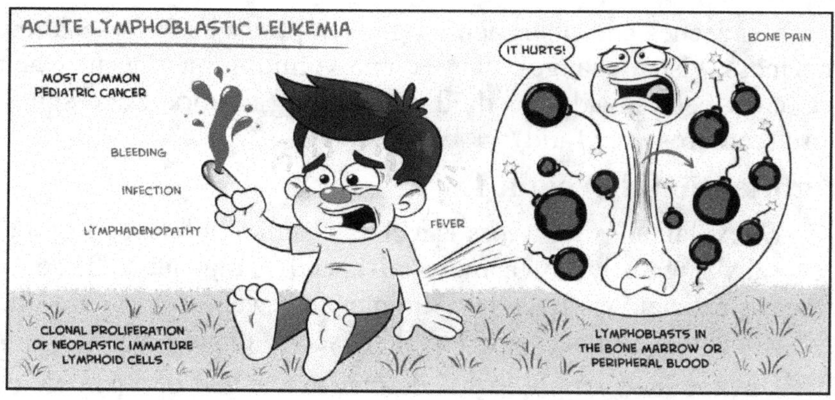

With T cell ALL, enlargement of the thymus gland, which lies behind the breastbone and in front of the trachea, may compress the trachea and lead to difficulty breathing.

Compression of the large vein returning blood from the upper body to the heart (the superior vena cava) may cause symptoms referred to superior vena cava syndrome. This can include marked swelling of the face, neck, upper arms, and upper chest.

Chronic Lymphocytic Leukemia (CLL)

The first symptom of chronic lymphocytic leukemia is often enlarged, painless lymph nodes in the neck, armpit, and groin. Other symptoms may come on very gradually and can include what is known as the "B symptoms," including fevers, chills, night sweats, and weight loss.

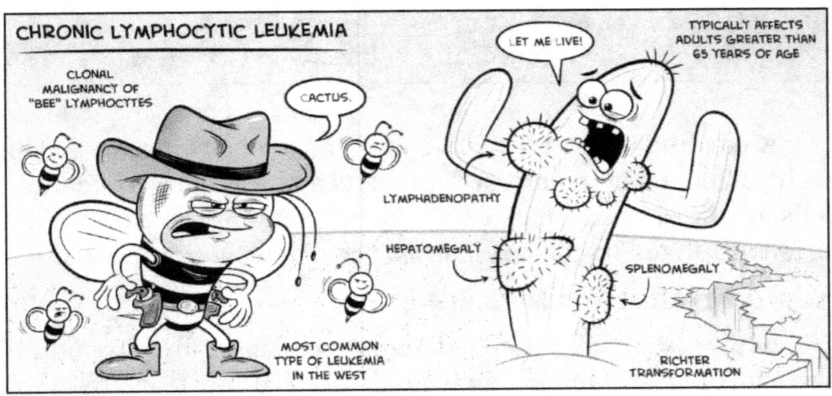

In around 5 percent of CLL diagnoses, the disease will transform into an aggressive lymphoma, known as Richter syndrome, characterized by widespread lymphadenopathy and the development of white blood cell tumors in multiple parts of the body.

Acute Myeloid Leukemia (AML)

Acute myeloid leukemia, like ALL, often comes on rapidly with the symptoms discussed above. AML is somewhat unique in that the immature white blood cells (blast cells) can clog blood vessels, something called leukostasis. This can result in symptoms similar to a stroke with visual changes or weakness of one side of the body. Greenish-tinged rashes called chloromas may occur due to the spread of AML cells under the skin.

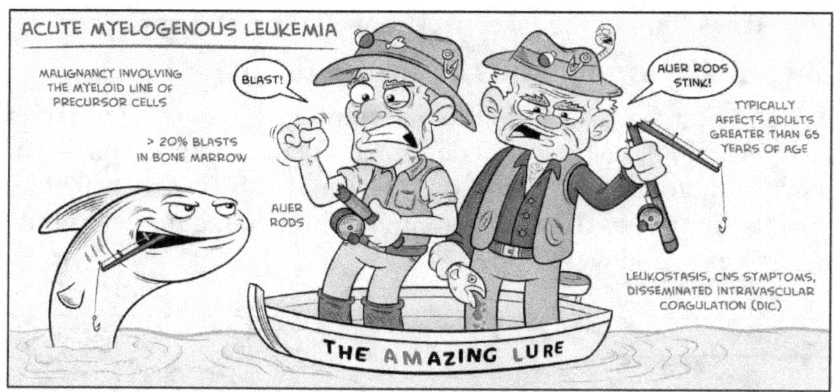

A condition called Sweet's syndrome may also occur. ☐ This is characterized by recurrent fevers and a build-up of white blood cells in the dermal layer of the skin, resulting in painful skin lesions scattered on the head, arms, neck, and chest.

Acute Promyelocytic Leukemia

Acute promyelocytic leukemia accounts for around 10 percent of AML cases and is distinctive in that the most prominent symptoms usually involve both excessive bleeding and excessive blood clotting. This may include nosebleeds, heavy periods, and bruising, but also leg and calf pain and swelling (due to deep vein thrombosis) and the sudden onset of chest pain and shortness of breath that can accompany pulmonary emboli (blood clots that break off in the legs and travel to the lungs).

Chronic Myeloid Leukemia (CML)

Chronic myeloid leukemia is most often suspected before any symptoms are present when the results of a complete blood count (CBC) are abnormal. Even after diagnosis, people with CML may have few if any symptoms for months or years before the leukemia cells begin to grow more quickly and make themselves known.

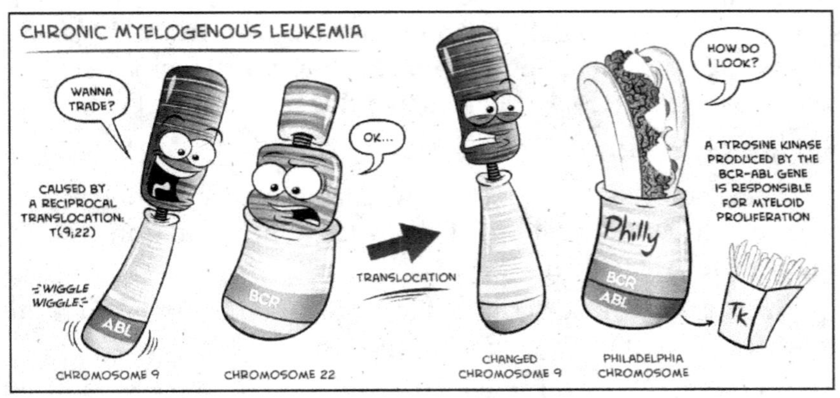

Chronic Myelomonocytic Leukemia (CMML)

Chronic myelomonocytic leukemia often affects many parts of the body, not just the bone marrow. Collections of monocytes in the spleen lead to enlargement (splenomegaly) which can cause pain in the left upper abdomen and fullness with eating. Collections of monocytes can cause enlargement of the liver (hepatomegaly) resulting in pain in the right upper abdomen as well.

Complications

There are many possible complications of leukemia, several of which are related to deficiency of the different types of white blood cells. A few of the more common concerns include:

Severe Infections

A reduced level of white blood cells reduces the body's ability to fight infections, and even relatively minor infections may become life-threatening. Infections such as urinary tract infections, pneumonia, and skin infections can rapidly progress to sepsis and septic shock (a widespread infection often accompanied by a drop in blood pressure and reduced level of consciousness).

During leukemia treatment, the suppression of the immune system can allow certain microorganisms to thrive and become life-threatening, including the chickenpox virus (herpes zoster), cytomegalovirus (CMV), and Aspergillus.

Serious Bleeding

While bleeding is common when the platelet count is low, bleeding in certain regions of the body can be life-threatening. Such instances include:

Intracranial hemorrhage: Bleeding into the brain can result in the rapid onset of confusion or unconsciousness.

Pulmonary hemorrhage: Bleeding in the lungs may result in severe shortness of breath and coughing up blood.

Gastrointestinal hemorrhage: Bleeding into the stomach and/or intestines can result in vomiting large amounts of blood and a rapid drop in blood pressure.

When to See a Doctor

It's important to see a doctor if you develop any of the symptoms above, or if you are just not feeling right. Trust your intuition. Because many of the symptoms of leukemia are non-specific, they could be indications of another serious condition as well.

Some symptoms, such as new onset severe headaches, other neurological symptoms, or drenching night sweats, should be addressed right away.

Others, such as swollen lymph nodes in the neck, should be evaluated if they persist—even if you think there is a logical explanation. Since acute lymphocytic leukemia often lacks symptoms early on, seeing a physician for a regular physical and blood tests is also important.

How Leukemia Is Diagnosed

Making an accurate diagnosis of leukemia is important in choosing the best treatment options. Testing often begins with a complete blood count and peripheral smear. A bone marrow aspiration and biopsy are also done with most types of leukemia.

Additional tests are then performed to look for surface markers on the cells (flow cytometry) as well as genetic changes (cytogenetic testing.) With some leukemias, a lumbar puncture (spinal tap), or lymph node biopsy may be perused as well.

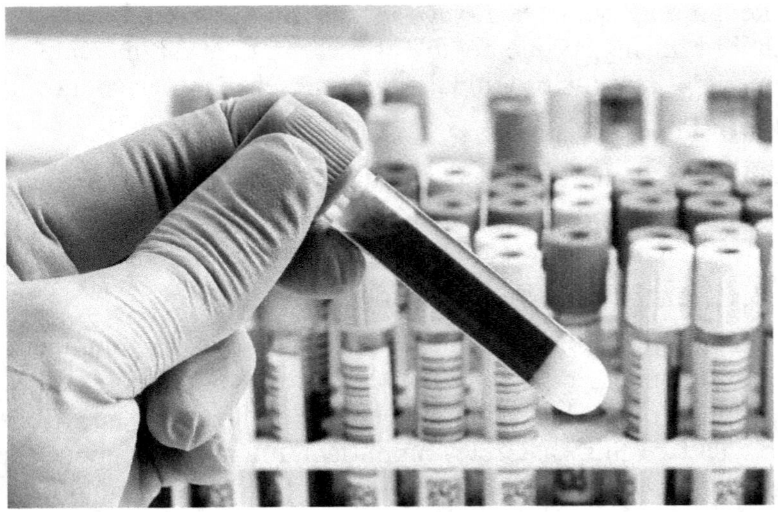

The cancer, if detected, is then staged based on factors such as symptoms, the subtype of leukemia, the number of abnormal cells in the blood or bone marrow, and more.

When talking about leukemia diagnosis, it's important to remember that leukemia is not one disease or even four diseases. Rather, there are many different variations.

Two leukemias that appear identical under the microscope may behave very differently, and some of the tests below may help to distinguish some of the differences.

Physical Exam and History

The history and physical examination are the starting point in the diagnosis of leukemia and what often prompts doctors to order further testing studies, but they cannot be used alone to make the diagnosis.

If leukemia is suspected, your doctor will ask about any symptoms of leukemia and risk factors for the disease that you may have. A physical examination may reveal signs that leukemia may be present, such as swelling of lymph nodes, pale skin, or bruising. While notable if present, they can indicate other concerns. Your doctor will take their presence into account.

Blood Tests

Both a complete blood count and peripheral smear, simple blood tests, can give important clues as to the diagnosis and type of leukemia, and guide further evaluation.

C.B.C. and Peripheral Blood Smear

A complete blood count (CBC) measures the numbers of each of the major types of blood cells made by the bone marrow: the white blood cells, red blood cells, and platelets. The CBC can also yield results that relay important information about these cells, such as whether the red blood cells are large or small.

While there is often an increase in white blood cells with leukemia, with acute leukemia there is sometimes a decrease in all of the types of blood cells, a condition referred to as pancytopenia.

A peripheral smear is a very important test when considering the diagnosis of leukemia. In a peripheral smear, a sample of blood is spread on a microscope slide and dye is added. The smear is then evaluated under a microscope.

A CBC can determine if a white blood cell count is low or high, but doesn't give enough information about the type of white blood cells that are increased or decreased.

It also doesn't tell a doctor whether there are immature white blood cells called "blasts" in the peripheral blood—cells that are normally only found in significant numbers in the bone marrow.

A peripheral smear can answer these questions by allowing technicians and doctors to directly observe the cells under the microscope.

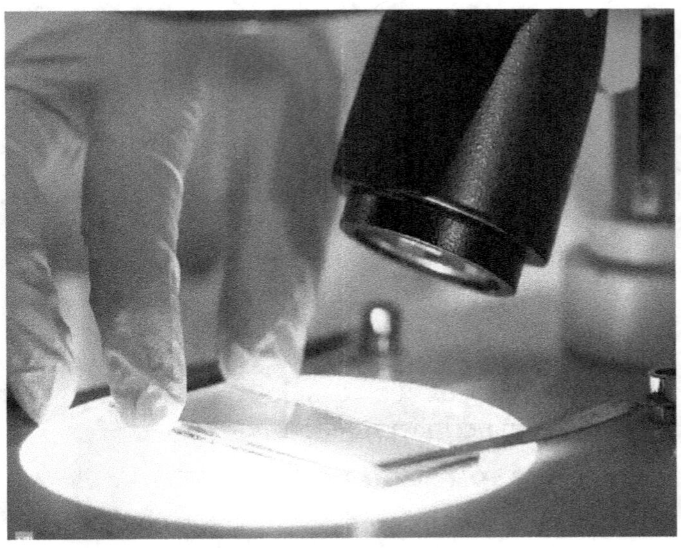

Typical findings (these can vary) on a CBC and blood smear for the four main types of leukemia include:

Disease	CBC Results	Blood Smear Results
Acute Myelogenous Leukemia (AML)	Lower than normal amounts of red cells and platelets	Many immature white cells, and sometimes the presence of Auer rods
Acute Lymphocytic Leukemia (ALL)	Lower than normal amounts of red cells and platelets	Many immature white cells
Chronic Myelogenous Leukemia (CML)	·Red blood cell count may be high and platelet count may be high or low ·White blood cell count may be very high ·Increased number of mature looking lymphocytes	·May show some immature white cells ·Mainly high numbers of fully mature white blood cells
Chronic Lymphocytic Leukemia (CLL)	·Red cells and platelets may or may not be decreased ·White blood cell count may be very high (over 20,000 cells/mm3 and sometimes over 100,000 cells/mm3)	·Little or no immature white cells ·Possibly fragments of red cells

Some of the tests discussed below, such as cytochemistry, may also be done on peripheral blood.

Bone Marrow Aspiration and Biopsy

Bone marrow aspiration and biopsy from the iliac crest

With most types of leukemia, blood tests are not enough to conclusively dignosis the disease, and a bone marrow aspiration and biopsy are done. (With CLL, the diagnosis can sometimes be made based on the blood tests above, but a bone marrow can still be helpful in determining how advanced the cancer is.) The bone marrow is the source of the cancer cells in leukemia and all of the blood cells found in the peripheral blood.

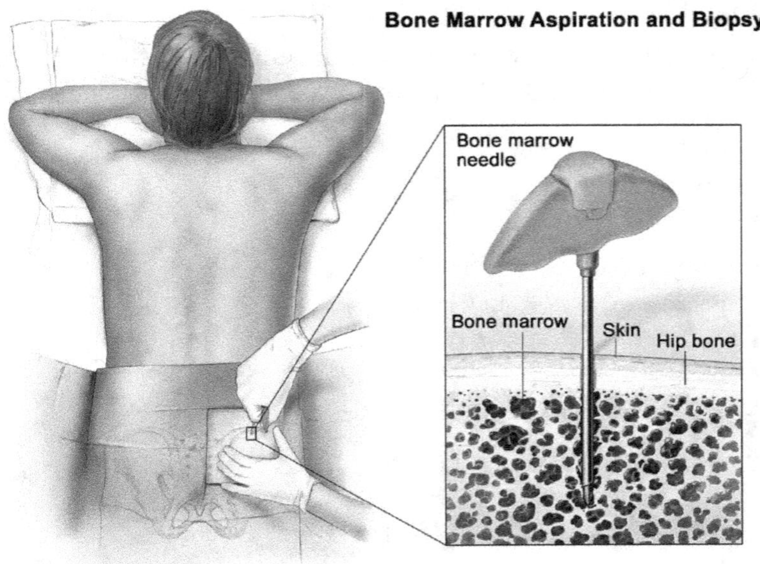

With a bone marrow aspiration, a long, thin needle is inserted into the bone marrow in the hip (or sometimes the breastbone) after numbing the skin locally with lidocaine. After a sample of the bone marrow is aspirated, a biopsy sample is also taken.

In normal bone marrow, between 1 percent and 5 percent of cells are blast cells, or the immature white blood cells that mature into those normally found in the blood.

A diagnosis of ALL can be made if at least 20% of the cells are blasts (lymphoblasts). With AML, a diagnosis can be made if there are less than 20% blasts (myeloblasts) if a specific chromosome change is also found.

In addition to looking at the number of different cells present in the bone marrow, doctors also look at the pattern of the cells.

For example, with CLL, the prognosis of the disease is better if the cancer cells are found in groups (nodular or interstitial pattern) than if they are found diffusely scattered around the bone marrow.

The ratio of leukemia cells to healthy blood-forming cells can be significant in the diagnostic process.

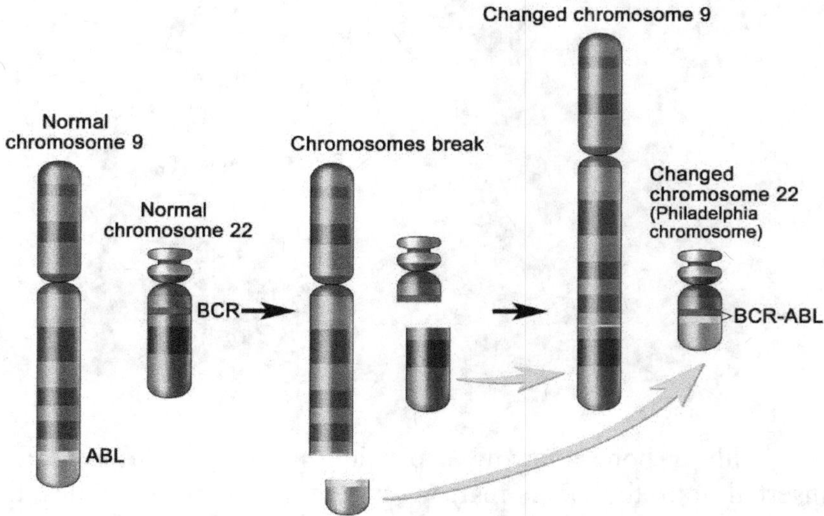

Cytochemistry

Cytochemistry looks at how the cells in the bone marrow take up certain stains and can be helpful in distinguishing ALL from AML. Tests can include both flow cytometry and immunohistochemistry.

In flow cytometry, the bone marrow cells (or peripheral blood cells) are coated with antibodies to look for the presence of certain proteins found on the surface of the cells. The antibodies will stick to these proteins and can be detected by the light they give off when a laser is introduced.

Immunohistochemistry is similar, but instead of using a laser to look for light given off by antibody-marked proteins, they can be seen under the microscope due to a color change.

This process of looking for unique proteins on the surface of cells is referred to as immunophenotyping. In genetics, genotype refers to the characteristics of a gene, whereas phenotype describes physical characteristics (such as blue eyes). Different types of leukemia differ in these phenotypes.

With acute leukemias (both ALL and AML), these studies can be helpful in determining the subtype of the disease, and with ALL, can determine if the leukemia involves T cells or B cells.

In addition, these tests can be very helpful in confirming a diagnosis of CLL (by looking for proteins called ZAP-70 and CD38).

Flow cytometry can also be used to determine the amount of DNA in leukemia cells, which can be helpful in planning treatment. ALL cells that have more DNA than an average cell tend to respond better to chemotherapy.

Chromosome and Gene Studies

Leukemia cells very often have changes in the chromosomes or genes found in the DNA of each cell. Each of our cells normally has 46 chromosomes, 23 from each parent, that contain many genes. Some studies look primarily at chromosomal changes, whereas others look for changes in specific genes.

Cytogenetics

Cytogenetics involves viewing the chromosomes of cancer cells under the microscope and looking for abnormalities.

Due to the method by which this is done (the cancer cells need time to be grown in the lab after being retrieved), the results of these studies are often not available for two to three weeks after a bone marrow biopsy is done.

Chromosomal changes that may be seen in the leukemia cells include:

- **Deletions:** Part of a chromosome is missing.

- **Translocations:** Pieces of two chromosomes are exchanged. This may be a complete exchange, in which pieces of DNA are simply swapped between two chromosomes, or a partial one. For example, DNA may be swapped between chromosomes 9 and 22. Chromosome translocations are very common in leukemia, occurring in up to 50 percent of these cancers.

- **Inversion:** Part of a chromosome remains present, but is turned around (as if a piece of a puzzle is removed and replaced, but backward).

- **Addition or duplication:** Extra copies of all or part of a chromosome are found.

- **Trisomy:** There are three copies of one of the chromosomes, rather than two.

In addition to further defining the type of leukemia, cytogenetics can help with planning treatment. For example, in ALL, leukemia cells that have more than 50 chromosomes respond better to treatment.

Fluorescent In Situ Hybridization (FISH)

Fluorescent in situ hybridization (FISH) is a procedure that uses special dyes to look for changes in chromosomes that can't be detected under the microscope, or changes in specific genes.

With chronic myelogenous leukemia (CML), this test can look for pieces of the BCR/ABL1 fusion gene (Philadelphia chromosome).

Roughly 95% of people with CML will have this shortened chromosome 22, but the other 5% will still have the abnormal BCR/ABL1 fusion gene on further testing. The Philadelphia chromosome is also an important finding with ALL.

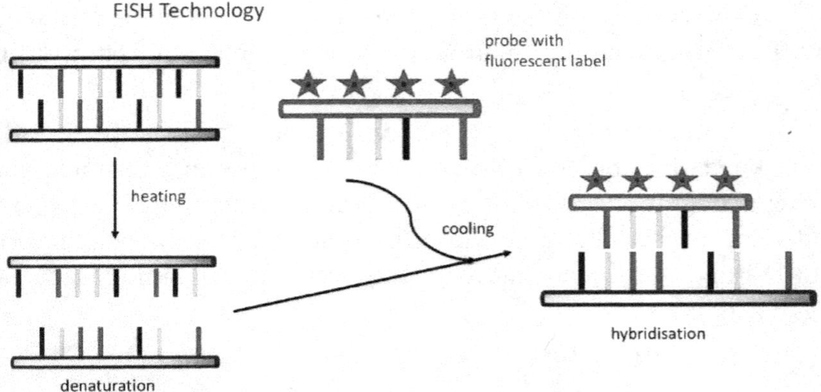

With CLL, cytogenetics is less helpful, and FISH and PCR are more important in finding genetic changes. There are many genetic abnormalities that may be seen in these studies, including deletions in the long arm of chromosome 13 (in half of the people with the disease), an extra copy of chromosome 12 (trisomy 12), deletions in the 17th and 11th chromosome, and specific mutations in genes such as NOTCH1, SF3B1, and more.

Polymerase Chain Reaction (PCR)

Like FISH, polymerase chain reaction (PCR) can find changes in chromosomes and genes that can't be seen through cytogenetics. PCR is also helpful in finding changes that are present in just a few, but not all, of the cancer cells.

PCR is very sensitive in finding the BCR/ABL gene, even when other signs of CML aren't found on chromosome testing.

Other Procedures

In addition to evaluating white blood cells in the blood and bone marrow, other procedures are sometimes done.

Lumbar Puncture (Spinal Tap)

With some types of leukemia, a spinal tap (lumbar puncture) may be done to look for the presence of leukemia cells that have spread into the fluid surrounding the brain and spinal cord.

☐It may be done for those with ALL, as well as people with AML who have any neurological symptoms suggesting this spread.

In a lumbar puncture, a person lies on a table on their side with knees up and head down. After cleaning and numbing the area, a doctor inserts a long thin needle into the lower back, between the vertebrae, and into the space surrounding the spinal cord. Fluid is then withdrawn and sent to a pathologist to be analyzed.

Lymph Node Biopsy

Lymph node biopsies, in which part or all of a lymph node are removed, are done infrequently with leukemia.☐ A lymph node biopsy may be done with CLL if large lymph nodes are present, or if it's thought that CLL may have transformed into a lymphoma.

Imaging

Imaging tests are not usually used as a diagnostic method for leukemia, as blood-related cancers like leukemia don't often form tumors. It may be helpful, however, in staging some leukemias, such as CLL.

X-Rays

X-rays, such as a chest X-ray or bone X-ray are not used to diagnose leukemia, but may give the first signs that something is wrong. An X-ray may show enlargement of lymph nodes or thinning of bones (osteopenia).

Computed Tomography (CT Scan)

A CT scan uses a series of X-rays to create a 3-dimensional picture of the inside of the body. CT may be helpful in looking at nodes in the chest or other regions of the body, as well as noting enlargement of the spleen or liver.

Magnetic Resonance Imaging (MRI)

An MRI uses magnets to create a picture of the inside of the body and does not involve radiation. It may be helpful in leukemias that involve the brain or spinal cord.

Positron Emission Tomography (PET/CT or PET/MRI)

In a PET scan, radioactive glucose is injected into the body, where it is taken up by cells that are more metabolically active (such as cancer cells). PET is more helpful with solid tumors than with leukemia, but may be helpful with some chronic leukemias, especially when there is concern about transformation into a lymphoma.

Differential Diagnosis

There are some diseases that, at least with initial testing, may resemble leukemia. Some of these include:

Certain viral infections: For example, the Epstein-Barr virus (the cause of infectious mononucleosis), cytomegalovirus, and HIV may cause an elevated number of atypical lymphocytes on blood tests.

Myelodysplastic syndromes: These are diseases of the bone marrow that have a predilection for developing into AML and are sometimes referred to as preleukemia.

Myeloproliferative disorders: Conditions such as polycythemia vera, essential thrombocytosis, primary myelofibrosis, and more may resemble leukemia prior to performance of the in-depth testing methods above.

Aplastic anemia: A condition in which the bone marrow stops making all of the types of blood cells.

Staging

Once leukemia has been confirmed, it must be staged. Staging refers to the system used by doctors to categorize a cancer. Determining the stage of a cancer, in general, can help doctors select the most appropriate treatment as well as estimate the prognosis of the disease.

Staging differs between the different types of leukemia. Since many leukemias do not form solid masses, staging (with the exception of CLL) is very different from that of solid tumors such as breast cancer or lung cancer.

A number of studies may be taken into consideration in assigning a stage, such as the number of immature white blood cells found in the blood or bone marrow, tumor markers, chromosome studies, and more.

When looking at staging, it's again important to note that leukemia is a wide range of diseases. Two people with the same kind of leukemia and the same stage may have very different responses to therapy, as well as different prognoses.

Chronic Lymphocytic Leukemia (CLL)

For chronic lymphocytic leukemia, there are a number of different staging systems that may be used. Most common is the Rai system. In this system, leukemias are given a stage between stage 0 and stage 4 based on the presence of several findings:

- High numbers of lymphocytes
- Enlarged lymph nodes
- An enlarged liver and/or spleen
- Anemia
- Low levels of platelets

Based on these stages, the cancers are then separated into low, intermediate, and high-risk categories.

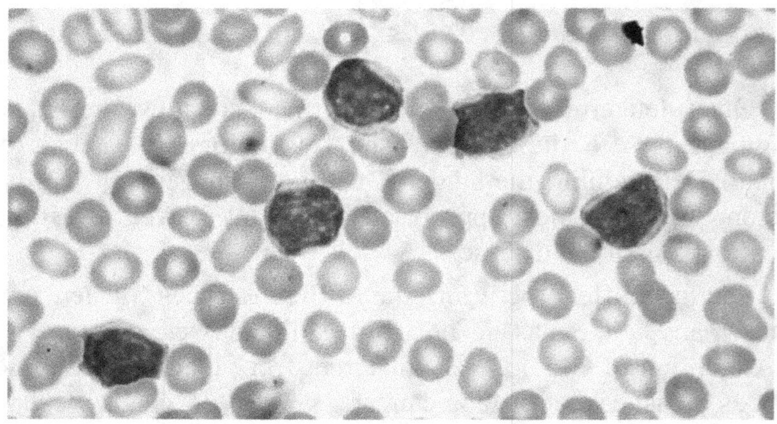

In contrast, the Binet system used in Europe separates these leukemias into only three stages:

Stage A: Less than 3 lymph nodes

Stage B: Greater than 3 affected lymph nodes

Stage C: Any number of lymph nodes, but combined with either anemia or a low level of platelets.

Acute Lymphocytic Leukemia (ALL)

For acute lymphocytic leukemia, staging is different, as the disease does not form tumor masses that extend incrementally from an original tumor.

ALL will likely spread to other organs even before it is detected, so rather than using traditional staging methods, physicians often factor in the subtype of ALL and the person's age.

This usually involves cytogenetic tests, flow cytometry, and other lab tests.

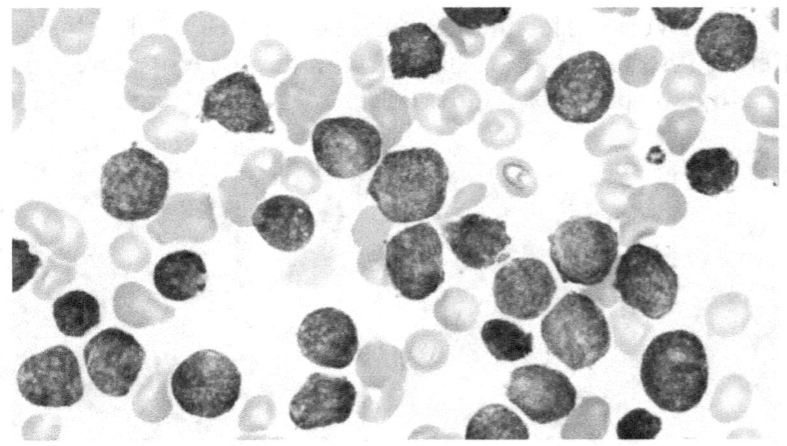

Rather than using stages (those used in the past are largely obsolete), ALL is more often defined by the "phases" of the disease. These include:

- Untreated ALL
- ALL in remission
- Minimal residual disease
- Refractory ALL
- Relapsed (recurrent) ALL

Acute Myelogenous Leukemia (AML)

Similar to ALL, acute myelogenous leukemia is usually not detected until it has spread to other organs, and so traditional cancer staging is not applicable. Staging is determined by characteristics such as the subtype of the leukemia, a person's age, and more.

An older staging system, the French-American-British (FAB) classification, classified AML into eight subtypes, M0 through M7, based on the appearance of the cells under the microscope.

The World Health Organization (WHO) developed a different system for AML staging with the hope of more closely predicting the prognosis of the disease.

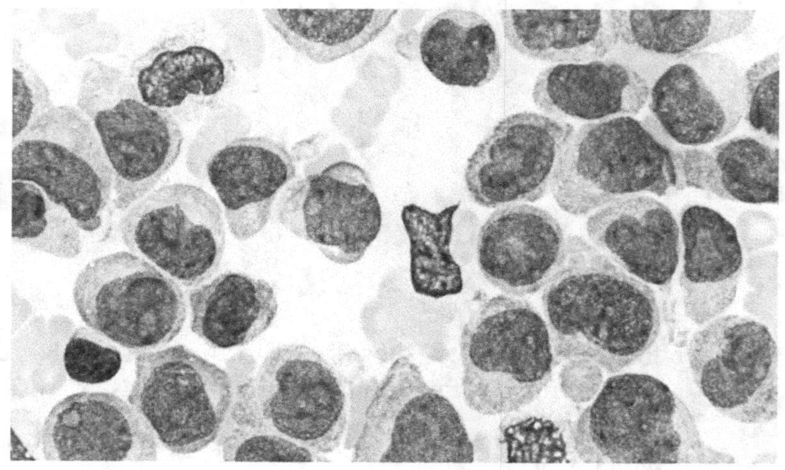

In this system, these leukemias are separated out by characteristics such as chromosomal abnormalities in the cells (some chromosome changes are associated with a better-than-average prognosis, while others are associated with poorer outcomes), whether the cancer arose after previous chemotherapy or radiation (secondary cancers), those related to Down syndrome, and more.

Chronic Myelogenous Leukemia (CML)

For chronic myeloid leukemia the presence of an increased number of mature cells belonging to the myeloid lineage (like neutrophils) is common. Staging is determined based on the number of immature myeloid cells at different stages of maturation:

Chronic phase: In this earliest stage, there are less than 10 percent blasts in the blood or bone marrow and symptoms are either mild or absent. People in the chronic phase of CML usually respond well to treatment.

Accelerated phase: In the next phase, 10 percent to 20 percent of the cells in the blood or bone marrow are blasts. Symptoms become more pronounced, particularly fever and weight loss. Testing may reveal new chromosomal changes in addition to the Philadelphia chromosome. People in the accelerated phase of CML may not respond to treatment.

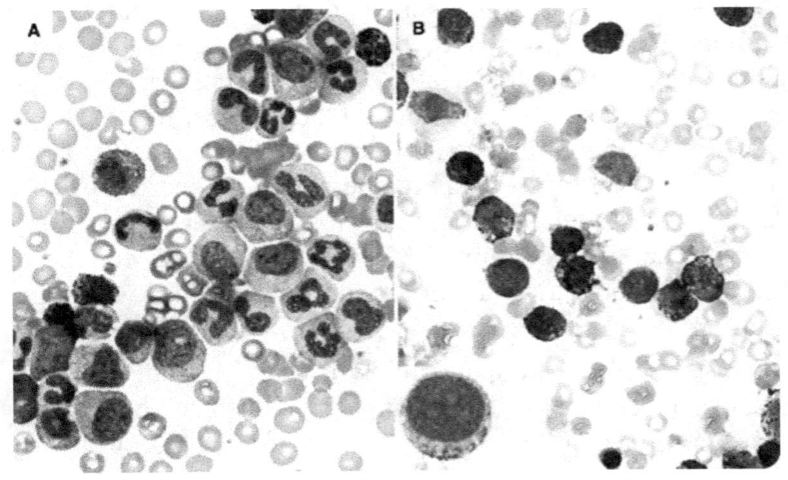

Blast phase (aggressive phase): In the blast phase of CML, more than 20 percent of the cells in the blood or bone marrow are blasts, and blast cells may also spread to areas of the body outside of the bone marrow. During this phase, symptoms include fatigue, fever, and an enlarged spleen (blast crisis).

How Leukemia Is Treated

The treatment for leukemia depends on many factors including the type and subtype of the disease, the stage, a person's age, and general health. Since leukemia is a cancer of blood cells, that travel throughout the body, local treatments such as surgery and radiation therapy are used infrequently. Instead, options such as aggressive chemotherapy, bone marrow/stem cell transplant, targeted therapy (tyrosine kinase inhibitors), monoclonal antibodies, immunotherapy, and others may be used alone or in combination. Even a period of watchful waiting may be appropriate in some cases.

Most people with leukemia will have a team of medical professionals caring for them, with a specialist in blood disorders and cancer (a hematologist/oncologist) leading the group.

The treatments for leukemia, especially acute leukemia, very often cause infertility. For this reason, people who may wish to have a child in the future should discuss fertility preservation before treatment begins.

Approaches by Disease Type

Before discussing the different types of treatments, it's helpful to understand common initial approaches to treatment for the different types of leukemia. You may find it useful to zero in on the type you have been diagnosed with, then jump ahead to the in-depth descriptions of each option.

Acute Lymphocytic Leukemia (ALL)

With acute lymphocytic leukemia (ALL), treatment of the disease can take several years. It begins with induction treatment and with the goal of remission. Consolidation chemotherapy is then given (several cycles) to address any remaining cancer cells and reduce the risk of relapse. Alternatively, some people may receive a hematopoietic stem cell transplant (though less commonly than with AML).

After consolidation therapy, maintenance chemotherapy is given (usually a lower dose) to further reduce the risk of relapse, with the goal being long-term survival. If leukemia cells are found in the central nervous system, chemotherapy is given directly into the spinal fluid (intrathecal chemotherapy). Radiation therapy may also be used if leukemia has spread to the brain, spinal cord, or skin. For those who have Philadelphia chromosome-positive ALL, the targeted therapy asparaginase may also be used.

Unfortunately, chemotherapy drugs do not penetrate well into the brain and spinal cord due to the presence of the blood-brain barrier, a tight network of capillaries that limits the ability of toxins (such as chemotherapy) to enter the brain. For this reason, many people are given preventive treatment to prevent leukemia cells from remaining behind in the central nervous system.

Acute Myelogenous Leukemia (AML)

Similar to the treatment of ALL, treatment for acute myelogenous leukemia (AML) usually begins with induction chemotherapy. After remission is achieved, further chemotherapy may be given, or, for people with a high risk of relapse, stem cell transplantation. Among the treatments for leukemia, those for AML tend to be the most intense and suppress the immune system to the greatest degree. Those over age 60 may be treated with less intense chemotherapy or palliative care, depending on the subtype of leukemia and general health.

Acute promyelocytic leukemia (APL) is treated with additional medications and has a very good prognosis.

Chronic lymphocytic leukemia

In the early stages of chronic lymphocytic leukemia (CLL), a period of no treatment referred to a watchful waiting is often the best "treatment option." This is often the best choice even if the white blood cell count is very high. If certain symptoms, physical findings, or changes in blood tests develop, treatment is often started with a combination of chemotherapy and a monoclonal antibody.

Chronic Myelogenous Leukemia

With chronic myelogenous leukemia (CML), tyrosinase kinase inhibitors (TKIs, a type of targeted therapy) have revolutionized the treatment of the disease and resulted in a dramatic improvement in survival over the past two decades. These drugs target the BCR-ABL protein that causes the cancer cells to grow. For those who develop resistance to two or more of these drugs, a newer chemotherapy drug was approved in 2012. Pegylated interferon (a type of immunotherapy) may be used for those who do not tolerate TKIs.

In the past, hematopoietic stem cell transplant was the treatment of choice for CML, but is used less commonly now and primarily in younger people with the disease.

Watchful Waiting

Most leukemias are treated aggressively when diagnosed, with the exception of CLL. Many people with this type of leukemia do not require treatment in the early stages of the disease, and a period of watchful waiting or active surveillance is considered a viable standard treatment option.

Watchful waiting does not mean the same thing as foregoing treatment and does not reduce survival when used appropriately. Instead, blood counts are done every few months, and treatment is initiated if constitutional symptoms (fever, night sweats, fatigue, weight loss greater than 10 percent of body mass), progressive fatigue, progressive bone marrow failure (with a low red blood cell or platelet count), painfully enlarged lymph nodes, a significantly enlarged liver and/or spleen, or a very high white blood cell count arise.

Chemotherapy

Chemotherapy is the mainstay of treatment for acute leukemias and is often combined with a monoclonal antibody for CLL. It may also be used for CML that has become resistant to targeted therapy.

Chemotherapy works by eliminating rapidly dividing cells such as cancer cells, but can also affect normal cells that divide rapidly, such as those in the hair follicles. It is most often given as combination chemotherapy (two or more drugs), with different drugs working at different places in the cell cycle.

The chemotherapy drugs chosen and the way in which they are used differs depending on the type of leukemia being treated.

Induction Chemotherapy

Induction chemotherapy is often the first therapy that is used when a person is diagnosed with acute leukemia. The goal of this treatment is to reduce the level of leukemia cells in the blood to undetectable levels. This does not mean that the cancer is cured, but only that it can't be detected when looking at a blood sample.

The other goal of induction therapy is to reduce the number of cancer cells in the bone marrow so that normal production of the different types of blood cells can resume. Unfortunately, further treatment is needed after induction therapy so that the cancer does not recur.

With AML, a common induction therapy is called the 7+3 protocol. This includes three days of an anthracycline, either Idamycin (idarubicin) or Cerubidine (daunorubicin), along with seven days of a continuous infusion of Cytosar U or Depocyt (cytarabine). These drugs are often given through a central venous catheter in the hospital (people are usually hospitalized for the first four to six weeks of treatment). For younger people, the majority will achieve remission.

Chemotherapy Drugs

With ALL, chemotherapy usually includes a combination of four drugs:

- An anthracycline, usually either Cerubidine (daunorubicin) or Adriamycin (doxorubicin)
- Oncovin (vincristine)
- Prednisone (a corticosteroid)
- An asparaginase: Either Elspar or L-Asnase (asparaginase) or Pegaspargase (Peg asparaginase)

People with Philadelphia chromosome-positive ALL and those over age 60 may also be treated with a tyrosine kinase inhibitor, such as Sprycel (dasatinib). After remission is achieved, preventive treatment to the central nervous system is used to prevent leukemia cells from remaining in the brain and spinal cord.

With acute promyelocytic leukemia (APL), induction therapy also includes the medication ATRA (all-trans-retinoic acid), sometimes combined with Trisenox or ATO (arsenic trioxide).

While induction therapy often achieves a complete remission, further therapy is needed so that the leukemia does not recur.

Consolidation and Intensification Chemotherapy

With acute leukemias, options after induction chemotherapy and remission include either further chemotherapy (consolidation chemotherapy) or high-dose chemotherapy plus stem cell transplantation. With AML, the most common treatment is three to five courses of further chemotherapy, though, for people with high-risk disease, a stem cell transplant is often recommended. With ALL, consolidation chemotherapy is usually followed by maintenance chemotherapy, but a stem cell transplant may also be recommended for some people.

Maintenance Chemotherapy (for ALL)

With ALL, further chemotherapy after induction and consolidation chemotherapy is often needed to reduce the risk of relapse and to improve long-term survival.☐ Drugs used often include methotrexate or 6-MP (6-mercaptopurine).

Chemotherapy for CLL

When symptoms occur in CLL, usually a combination of the chemotherapy drug Fludara (fludarabine) with or without Cytoxan (cyclophosphamide) along with a monoclonal antibody such as Rituxan (rituximab) is recommended. As an alternative, the chemotherapy drug Treanda or Bendeka (bendamustine) may be used with a monoclonal antibody.

Chemotherapy for CML

The mainstay of treatment for CML is monoclonal antibodies, but chemotherapy may occasionally be recommended. Drugs such as Hydrea (hydroxyurea), Ara-C (cytarabine), Cytoxan (cyclophosphamide), Oncovin (vincristine), or Myleran (busulfan) may be used to lower a very high white blood cell count or enlarged spleen.

In 2012, a new chemotherapy drug—Synribo (omacetaxine)—was approved for CML that has progressed to the accelerated phase and has become resistant to two or more tyrosine kinase inhibitors or has the T3151 mutation.

Side Effects

Common side effects of chemotherapy can vary with the different drugs used, but may include:

- **Tissue damage:** Anthracyclines are vesicants and can cause tissue damage if they leak into the tissues surrounding the infusion site.

- **Bone marrow suppression:** Damage to rapidly dividing cells in the bone marrow often results in low levels of red blood cells (chemotherapy-induced anemia), white blood cells such as neutrophils (chemotherapy-induced neutropenia), and platelets (chemotherapy-induced thrombocytopenia). Due to a low white blood cell count, taking precautions to reduce the risk of infections is extremely important.

- **Hair loss:** Hair loss is common, not just what's on the top of the head, but the eyebrows, eyelashes, and pubic hair.

- **Nausea and vomiting:** While a feared side effect, medications to both treat and prevent chemotherapy-associated vomiting have reduced this significantly.

- **Mouth sores:** Mouth sores are common, though dietary changes, as well as mouth rinses, can improve comfort. Taste changes may also occur.

- **Red urine:** Anthracycline medications been coined the "red devils" for this common side effect. Urine may be bright red to orange in appearance, beginning shortly after the infusion and lasting for a day or so after it's complete. Though perhaps startling, it's not dangerous.

- **Peripheral neuropathy:** Numbness, tingling, and pain in a "stocking and glove" distribution (both the feet and the hands) may occur, especially with drugs such as Oncovin.

- **Tumor lysis syndrome:** The rapid breakdown of leukemia cells can result in a condition known as tumor lysis syndrome. Findings include high potassium, uric acid, blood urea nitrogen (BUN), and phosphate levels in the blood. Tumor lysis syndrome is less problematic than in the past, and is treated with intravenous fluids and medications to lower the uric acid level.

- **Diarrhea**

Since many people who develop leukemia are young and are expected to survive treatment, the late effects of treatment that may occur years or decades after treatment are of particular concern.

Potential long-term side effects of chemotherapy may include an increased risk of heart disease, secondary cancers, and infertility among others.

Targeted Therapy

Targeted therapies are medications that work by specifically targeting cancer cells or pathways involved in the growth and division of cancer cells. Unlike chemotherapy drugs, which can affect both cancer cells and normal cells in the body, targeted therapies focus on mechanisms that support the growth of a cancer specifically. For this reason, they may have fewer side effects than chemotherapy (but not always).

Unlike chemotherapy drugs that are cytotoxic (cause the death of cells), targeted therapies control the growth of cancer but do not kill cancer cells. While they may hold a cancer in check for years or even decades, as is often the case with CML, they are not a cure for cancer.

In addition to the targeted therapies mentioned below, there are a number of drugs that may be used for leukemia that has relapsed or leukemias that harbor specific genetic mutations.

Tyrosine Kinase Inhibitors (TKIs) for CML

Tyrosine inhibitors (TKIs) are medications that target enzymes called tyrosine kinases to interrupt the growth of cancer cells.

With CML, TKIs have revolutionized treatment and have vastly improved survival over the past two decades. Continued use of the drugs can often result in long-term remission and survival with CML. Medications currently available include:

- Gleevec (imatinib)
- Bosulif (bosutinib)

- Sprycel (dasatinib)
- Tasigna (nilotinib)
- Iclusig (ponatinib)

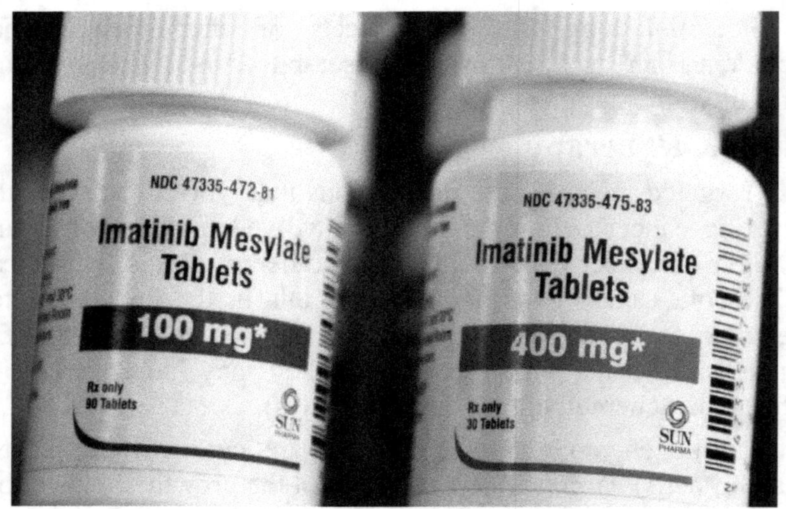

Kinase Inhibitors for ALL

With high-risk ALL, the TKIs Sprycel or Jakafi (ruxolitinib) may be used.

Kinase Inhibitors for CLL

In addition to monoclonal antibodies which are the mainstay of treatment, kinase inhibitors may be used for CLL. Drugs include:

- **Imbruvica (ibrutinib):** This drug that inhibits Bruton's tyrosine kinase may be effective for difficult-to-treat CLL.

- **Zydelig (idelalisib):** This drug blocks a protein (P13K) and may be used when other treatments are not working.

- **Venclextra (venetoclax):** This drug blocks a protein (BCL-2) and may be used second line to treat CLL.

Monoclonal Antibodies

Monoclonal antibodies are similar to the antibodies many people are familiar with that attack viruses and bacteria, but instead are man-made and designed to attack cancer cells.

For CLL, monoclonal antibodies are a mainstay of treatment, often combined with chemotherapy. These drugs target a protein (CD20) found on the surface of B cells. Drugs currently approved include:

- Rituxan (rituximab)
- Gazyva (obinutuzumab)
- Arzerra (ofatumumab)

These drugs can be very effective, though they do not work as well for people with a mutation or deletion in chromosome 17.

For refractory B cell ALL, the monoclonal antibodies Blincyto (blinatumomab) or Besponsa (inotuzumab) may be used.

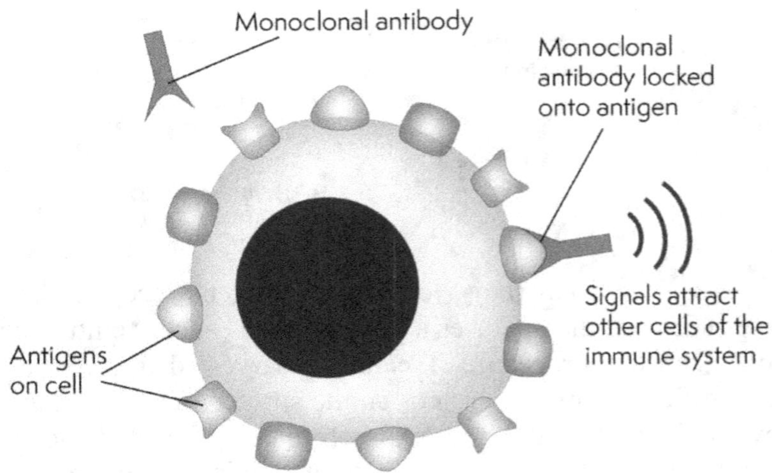

Proteasome Inhibitors

For refractory ALL in children, the proteasome inhibitor Velcade (bortezomib) may be used.

Immunotherapy

There is a wide range of treatments that fall under the general category of immunotherapy. These drugs work by using the immune system or principles of the immune system to fight cancer.

CAR T-Cell Therapy

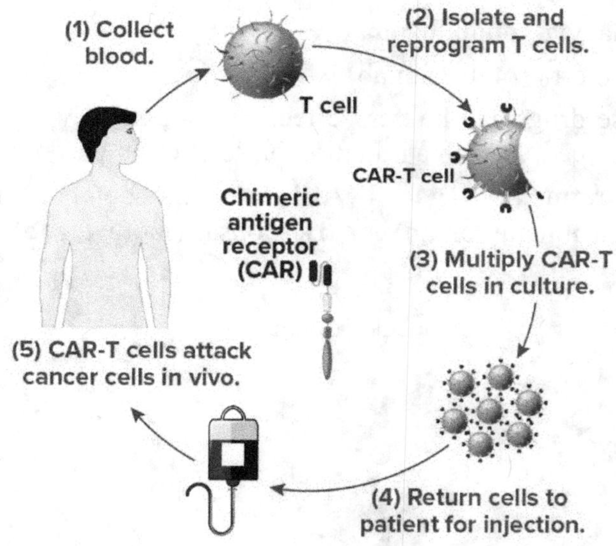

CAR T-cell therapy (chimeric antigen receptor T-cell therapy) or gene therapy uses a person's own cancer-fighting cells (T cells). In this procedure, T cells are harvested from the body and modified to target a protein on the surface of leukemia cells. They are then allowed to multiply before being injected back into the body, where they often eliminate leukemia cells within a few weeks.

In 2017, the drug **Kymriah** (tisagenlecleucel) received U.S. Food and Drug Administration (FDA) approval for children and young adults with B cell ALL or other types of ALL that have recurred.

Interferon

Interferons are substances made by the human body that function to control the growth and division of cancer cells, among other immune functions. In contrast to the CAR T-cell therapy, which is designed to attack particular markers on leukemia cells, interferons are non-specific and have been used in many settings from cancer to chronic infections. Interferon alpha, a man-made interferon, was once commonly used for CML, but is now used more often for people with CML who are intolerant of other treatments. It can be given by injection (either subcutaneously or intramuscularly) or intravenously, and is given for a long period of time.

Bone Marrow/Stem Cell Transplants

Hematopoietic cell transplants, or bone marrow and stem cell transplants, work by replacing the hematopoietic cells in the bone marrow that develop into the different types of blood cells. In these transplants, a person's bone marrow cells are destroyed. They are then replaced with donated cells that restock the bone marrow and eventually produce healthy white blood cells, red blood cells, and platelets.

Types

While bone marrow transplants (cells harvested from the bone marrow and injected) were once more common, peripheral blood stem cell transplants are now more so. Stem cells are harvested from the blood of a donor (in a procedure similar to dialysis) and collected. Medications are given to the donor prior to this procedure to increase the number of stem cells in the peripheral blood.

Types of hematopoietic cell transplants include:

- **Autologous transplants:** Transplants in which a person's own stem cells are used

- **Allogeneic transplants:** Transplants in which stem cells are derived from a donor, such as a sibling or unknown but matched donor

- **Transplants from umbilical cord blood**

- **Non-ablative stem cell transplant:** These transplants are less invasive "mini-transplants" that do not require obliterating the bone marrow prior to the transplant. Mini-transplants work by something called "graft versus malignancy" in which the donor cells help fight off the cancer cells, rather than by replacing the cells in the bone marrow.

Uses

A hematopoietic cell transplant may be used after induction chemotherapy with both AML and ALL, especially for high-risk disease. The goal of treatment with acute leukemia is long-term remission and survival. With CLL, stem cell transplantation may be used when other treatments do not control the disease. With CML, stem cell transplants were once the treatment of choice, but are now used much less often.

Non-ablative transplants may be used for people who would not tolerate the high-dose chemotherapy required for a traditional stem cell transplant (for example, people over the age of 50). They may also be used when a leukemia recurs after a previous stem cell transplant.

Phases of Stem Cell Transplants

Stem cell transplants have three distinct phases:

Induction: The induction phase is similar to that noted under chemotherapy for acute leukemias above and consists of using chemotherapy to reduce the white blood cell count and, if possible, induce a remission.

Conditioning: During this phase, high-dose chemotherapy and/or radiation therapy is used to destroy the bone marrow. In this phase, chemotherapy is used to essentially sterilize/obliterate the bone marrow so that no hematopoietic stem cells remain.

Transplantation: In the transplantation phase, the donated stem cells are given. Following transplantation, it usually takes from two to six weeks for the donated cells to grow in the bone marrow and produce functioning blood cells, what's known as engraftment.

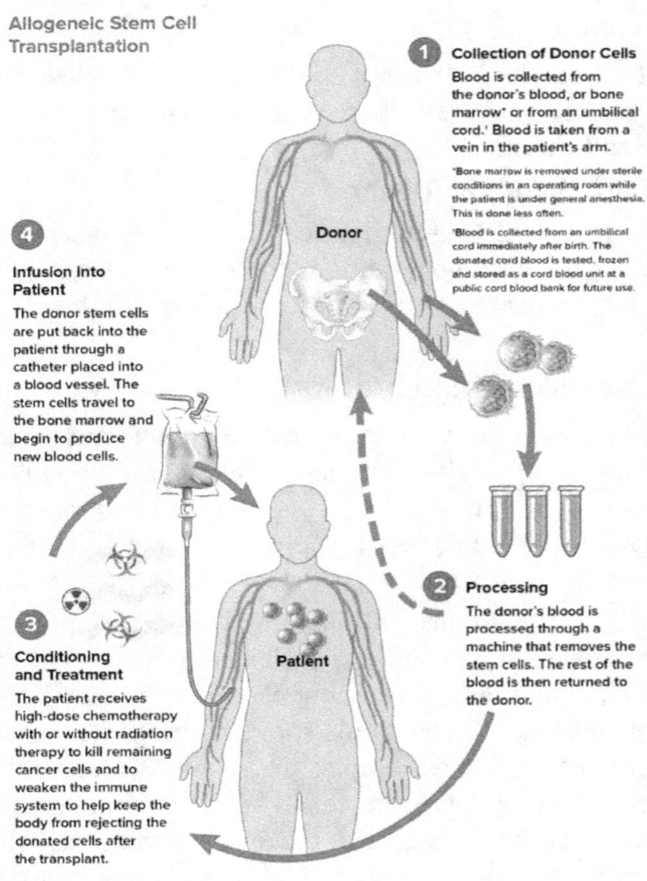

Side Effects and Complications

Stem cell transplants are major procedures and, though they can sometimes bring about a cure, have significant mortality (primarily due to the absence of infection-fighting cells between conditioning and the time it takes the donated cells to grow up in the marrow, when people have essentially no white blood cells left to fight infections). A few possible complications include:

Immunosuppression: As noted, a severely suppressed immune system is responsible for the relatively high mortality rate of this procedure.

Graft-versus-host disease: Graft-versus-host disease occurs when the donated cells attack a person's own cells and can be both acute and chronic.

Finding a Stem Cell Donor

For those considering as stem cell transplant, the oncologist will first want to check your siblings for a potential match. There are a number of resources available on how to find a donor, if needed.

Complementary Medicine

There are currently no alternative treatments that are effective in successfully treating leukemia, though some integrative cancer treatments such as meditation, prayer, yoga, and massage may help people cope with the symptoms of leukemia and its treatments.

While we often think of vitamins, minerals, and dietary supplements as relatively harmless, it's important to note that some vitamins may interfere with cancer treatments. This is easier to understand if you think about how cancer treatments work. Chemotherapy, for example, works by creating oxidative stress and damaging DNA in cells. While taking antioxidant preparations may be a healthful dietary practice for someone without cancer, there's a risk that using these same preparations may help "protect" cancer cells from the treatments designed to eliminate them.

While there has been some research that suggests that vitamin C may be helpful when combined with a class of medications called PARP inhibitors (which are not currently approved for leukemia), there have also been studies that suggest vitamin C supplementation makes chemotherapy less effective with leukemia.

The general uncertainty in this area is a good reminder to talk to your oncologist about any vitamins, dietary supplements, or over-the-counter medications you consider taking.

Clinical Trials

There are many different clinical trials in progress looking at more effective ways to treat leukemia or methods that have fewer side effects. With treatments for cancer rapidly improving, the National Cancer Institute recommends that people talk with their oncologist about the option of a clinical trial.

Some of the treatments being tested combine therapies mentioned above, whereas others are looking at unique ways to treat leukemia, including many next-generation drugs. The science is changing rapidly. For example, the first monoclonal antibody was only approved in 2002, and since then, second- and third-generation drugs have become available. Similar progress is being made with other types of targeted therapies and immunotherapy.

Alternative cancer treatments

We are fighting with cancer since the dawn of history. Every year we discover new diagnostic modalities, better radiotherapy techniques and lots of new chemotherapy drugs. But we have completely failed to defeat this disease called cancer. Think again, are we really going on the right path? Does conventional Medicine really targets upon the prime cause of cancer?

It's not that more effective alternative treatments for cancer don't exist — they most certainly do. It's just that the allopathic system isn't at all interested in divulging real cures. This is because their expensive therapies generate billions of dollars for the cancer industry.

Chemotherapy Doesn't Cure Cancer — It Causes It!

Chemotherapy does, in fact, kill cancer cells. But it also kills healthy cells, along with a patient's immune system and, really, anything else that crosses its path. At worst, such treatments kill patients more quickly than if they had chosen not to undergo them at all.

There's no money to be made in prescribing prevention advice like eating fewer chemicals and exercising more. The "bread and butter" of the cancer industry is unleashing the next, latest-and-greatest cancer drug. Not telling you how to avoid cancer in the first place.

Many people with cancer are interested in trying any treatment that may cure them safely, including complementary and alternative cancer treatments. There is growing evidence that these alternative cancer treatments give wonderful results. Here are some alternative cancer treatments that are very safe and effective.

- **Budwig Protocol -** *The best Alternative Treatment effective in all cancers and all stages with documented 90% success*
- Laetrile (Vitamin B-17) Therapy
- Gerson Therapy
- Dr. Simoncini Baking Soda Cancer Treatment
- High-dose vitamin C
- Frankincense Essential Oil Therapy
- Immunotherapy
- Hyperthermia
- Oxygen Therapy and Hyperbaric Chambers

Laetrile (Vitamin B-17) Therapy

Introduction

During 1950, after many years of research, a dedicated biochemist Dr. Ernest T. Krebs Jr., isolated a new vitamin from bitter apricot kernel that he called 'B-17' or 'Laetrile'. He conducted further lab animal and culture experiments to conclude that laetrile would be effective in the treatment of cancer. As the years rolled by, thousands became convinced that Krebs had finally found the treatment for all cancers. He proposed that cancer was caused by a deficiency of Vitamin B 17 (Laetrile, Amygdaline).

To prove that it was not toxic to humans he injected it into his own arm. As he predicted, there were no harmful or distressing side effects. The Laetrile had no harmful effect on normal cells but was deadly to cancer cells. Dr. Ernst Krebs stated that we need at least a minimum of 100 mg of B-17 or around 7 bitter apricot seeds to almost guarantee a cancer free life.

Nitriloside is a beta-cyanophoric glycosides, a large group of water-soluble, sugar-containing compounds found in a number of plants. Amygdalin is one of the most common nitrilosides. Laetrile is a partly man-made molecule and shares only part of the Amygdalin structure. Both Laetrile and Amygdalin have been promoted as "Vitamin B-17".

Laetrile stands for laevo-rotatory mandelonitrile beta-diglucoside. The "laevo" part references a purified form of B-17 that turns polarized light in a left-turning direction. Dr. Krebs, Jr. believed that only the left-rotating Laevo form was effective against cancer. So it's important to check the purity of your Laetrile.

How B-17 works (A tale of two enzymes)

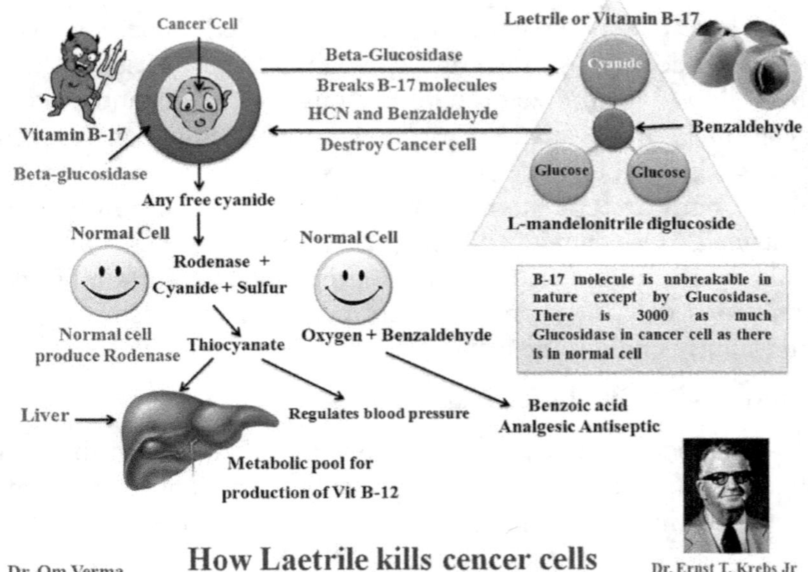

How Laetrile kills cencer cells

Laetrile, commonly known as Vitamin B-17 or Amygdalin, contains two units of Sugar, one of Benzaldehyde and one of Cyanide, all tightly locked within it. Everyone knows that cyanide can be highly toxic and even fatal if taken in sufficient quantity. However, as it is in locked state is completely inert and absolutely has no effect on living tissue. There is only one substance that can unlock this molecule and release the cyanide. That substance is an enzyme called beta-glucocidase, which we shall call the unlocking enzyme. When B-17 comes in contact with this enzyme, not only the cyanide is released but also Benzaldehyde which is highly toxic by itself. In fact, these two working together are at least 100 times more poisonous to cancer cell than either of them separately. The unlocking enzyme is not found to any dangerous degree anywhere in the body except at the cancer cell where it is present in great quantity. The result is that Vit B-17 is unlocked at the cancer cells becomes poisonous to the cancer cells and only to the cancer cells.

There is another important enzyme called Rodanese, which we shall identify as protecting enzyme. The reason is that it has the ability to neutralize cyanide by converting it instantly into the byproducts (thiocyanate) that actually are beneficial and essential for health. This enzyme is found in great quantities in every part of the body except the cancer cells which consequently is not protected. Here then is a biochemical process that destroys cancer cells while at the same time nourishing and sustaining non-cancerous cells. It is intricate and perfect mechanism of nature that simply couldn't be accidental.

Laetrile - Metabolic Therapy

Metabolic therapy is a non-toxic cancer treatment based on the use of Vitamin B- 17, proteolytic pancreatic enzymes, immuno-stimulants, and vitamin and mineral supplements.

There are three parts to this program:
1. Laetrile
2. Vitamins and enzymes
3. Diet

Phase I Metabolic - Program for the first 21 days

Laetrile

Amygdalin (Laetrile) is available in 500 mg. tablets and in vials (10 cc 3 Gm) for intravenous use. Both forms are used. Two vials of Laetrile are given IV three times weekly for three weeks with at least one day between injections (Mon., Wed., Fri.). Dose of Amygdalin Tablets 500 mg is 2 tab three times a day with meals on the days on which the patients do not receive the intravenous Laetrile. Thiocyanate levels in the blood can be measured during treatment. In general, the patients who do best are those in whom the thiocyanate level is between 1.2 and 2.5 Mg/DL (Philip E.Binzel   ).

Vitamins and Enzymes

Preven-Ca Caps - Preven-Ca is a comprehensive blend of potent herb and fruit extracts, designed to provide a broad Spectrum of Flavonoids with scientifically demonstrated Antioxidant activity and effectiveness. One capsule with each meal.

Vitamin B15 - One capsule three times a daily at the end of each meal.

Megazyme Forte (Proteolytic Enzymes) Three tablets two hours after each meal (9 daily).

Ester Vitamin C 1000 mg capsule - One capsule with each meal.

Shark Cartilage It has been said that Sharks are the healthiest creature on earth. Sharks are immune to practically every disease known to man. One capsules three times a daily with each meal.

Natural Vitamin E 400 iu - One gel with lunch and one with dinner.

AHCC (Active Hexose Correlated Compound) - Two capsules with each meal.

Multi Vitamin & Mineral Liquid - 1 oz (two tablespoons) once daily with a meal.

Vitamin A & E Emulsion - 5 drops in juice or water three times per day.

Barley Grass Juice - One teaspoon in juice three times per day.

Bitter apricot seeds - No more than 12 every 2 hours 6 times a day.

Dimethyl sulfoxide (DMSO) - DMSO is a by-product of the wood and paper industry. It is known for its ability to permeate living tissue and stimulate cellular processes.

Or Phase 1 Oral

Injectable Amygdalin is replaced with 500mg Amygdalin tablets. Binzel recommends 2 of these tablets with each meal for a total of 6 per day. Otherwise the ORAL Phase 1 includes the same materials as above.

Phase 2 Metabolic - Program for the next 3 months

It comprises the same materials as Phase 1 except that the dosages for the vitamin B-17 as well as the A&E Emulsion Drops change to the following:

Vitamin B-17 500 mg tablets: 1 tablet with each meal and one at bedtime.

Vitamin A & E emulsion drops: 10 drops in juice or water two times per day (suspend for 2 months after 3 months of use).

Diet

Consume those fruits (i.e. seeds), grains and nuts that are rich in laetrile. Consume salads with healthy dressings. For protein patient should consume whole grains including corn, beans, buckwheat, nuts, dried fruits. Real butter in small amounts is permitted. The patients are not permitted anything which contains white flour or white sugar. Take away all meat, all poultry, all fish, all eggs and milk from patients. Margarine is detrimental to good nutrition. No coffee is permitted.

Zinc acts as transport vehicle for laetrile in the body. If patient does not have sufficient zinc, laetrile will not get into the tissues of the body. That's why you should give a spoonful of pumpkin seeds along with bitter apricot kernels. The body will not rebuild any tissue without sufficient quantities of Vitamin C etc.

The Gerson Therapy

The Gerson Therapy is a natural treatment that activates the body's extraordinary ability to heal itself through an organic, plant-based diet, raw juices, coffee enemas and natural supplements.

With its whole-body approach to healing, the Gerson Therapy naturally reactivates your body's magnificent ability to heal itself – with no damaging side effects. This a powerful, natural treatment boosts the body's own immune system to heal cancer, arthritis, heart disease, allergies, and many other degenerative diseases. Dr. Max Gerson developed the Gerson Therapy in the 1930s, initially as a treatment for his own debilitating migraines, and eventually as a treatment for degenerative diseases such as skin tuberculosis, diabetes and, most famously, cancer.

An abundance of nutrients from copious amounts of fresh, organic juices are consumed every day, providing your body with a super-dose of enzymes, minerals and nutrients. These substances then break down diseased tissue in the body, while coffee enemas aid in eliminating toxins from the liver.

Throughout our lives our bodies are being filled with a variety of carcinogens and toxic pollutants. These toxins reach us through the air we breathe, the food we eat, the medicines we take and the water we drink. The Gerson Therapy's intensive detoxification regimen eliminates these toxins from the body, so that true healing can begin.

How the Gerson Therapy Works

The Gerson Therapy regenerates the body to health, supporting each important metabolic requirement by flooding the body with nutrients from about 15- 20 pounds of organically-grown fruits and vegetables daily. Most is used to make fresh raw juice, up to one glass every hour, up to 13 times per day. Raw and cooked solid foods are generously consumed. Oxygenation is usually more than doubled, as oxygen deficiency in the blood contributes to many degenerative diseases. The metabolism is also stimulated through the addition of thyroid, potassium and other supplements, and by avoiding heavy animal fats, excess protein, sodium and other toxins.

Degenerative diseases render the body increasingly unable to excrete waste materials adequately, commonly resulting in liver and kidney failure. The Gerson Therapy uses intensive detoxification to eliminate wastes, regenerate the liver, reactivate the immune system and restore the body's essential defenses – enzyme, mineral and hormone systems. With generous, high-quality nutrition, increased oxygen availability, detoxification, and improved metabolism, the cells – and the body – can regenerate, become healthy and prevent future illness.

Juicing

Fresh-pressed juice from raw foods provides the easiest and most effective way of providing high-quality nutrition. By juicing, patients can take in the nutrients and enzymes from nearly 15 pounds of produce every day, in a manner that is easy to digest and absorb.

Every day, a typical patient on the Gerson Therapy for cancer consumes up to thirteen glasses of fresh, raw carrot-apple and green leaf juices. These juices are prepared hourly from fresh, raw, organic fruits and vegetables, using a two-step juicer or a masticating juicer used with a separate hydraulic press.

The Gerson Therapy Diet

The Gerson Therapy diet is plant-based and entirely organic. The diet is naturally high in vitamins, minerals, enzymes, micro-nutrients, and extremely low in sodium, fats, and proteins. The following is a typical daily diet for a Gerson patient on the full therapy regimen:

- Thirteen glasses of fresh, raw carrot-apple and green-leaf juices prepared hourly from fresh, organic fruits and vegetables.
- Three full plant-based meals, freshly prepared from organically grown fruits, vegetables and whole grains. A typical meal will include salad, cooked vegetables, baked potatoes, Hippocrates soup and juice.
- Fresh fruit and vegetables available at all hours for snacking, in addition to the regular diet.

Supplements

All medications used in connection with the Gerson Therapy are classed as biologicals, materials of organic origin that are supplied in therapeutic amounts. The supplements used on the Gerson Therapy include:
- Potassium compound
- Lugol's solution
- Vitamin B-12
- Thyroid hormone
- Pancreatic Enzymes

Detoxification

Coffee enemas are the primary method of detoxification of the tissues and blood on the Gerson Therapy. Coffee enemas accomplish this essential task, assisting the liver in eliminating toxic residues from the body for good. Cancer patients on the Gerson Therapy may take up to 5 coffee enemas per day. The Gerson Therapy also utilizes castor oil to stimulate bile flow and enhance the liver's ability to filter blood.

Simoncini's Baking Soda Cancer Treatment

Dr. Tullio Simoncini is a medical doctor in Italy who has done more than anyone to explore the uses of the baking soda cancer treatment as an alternative cancer treatment. It is known that cancer creates and favors an acid environment and because of this, Dr. Simoncini and others have used sodium bicarbonate as an alkaline therapeutic agent.

The way that acidity seems to protect cancer is not fully understood. It seems that cytotoxic T-cells, which may attack cancer cells under normal conditions, are inactivated in an acid extracellular fluid. Also, the type of acidity that cancer produces, i.e., lactic acid, stimulates vascular endothelial growth factor and angiogenesis. This is like a highway project, which enables a tumor to build the blood vessels that it needs to bring the nutrients for it to survive. So the tumor creates an environment in which it can then exist comfortably.

Baking Soda's Alkalinity Fights Cancer's Acidity

At a pH of about 10, sodium bicarbonate is an antidote to this acidity. It can be used clinically in sterile, intravenous form. This is a liquid, sterile bicarbonate of soda. The baking soda cancer treatment is well-tolerated, even with frequent repeated dosing. Dr. Simonchini also injects soda bicarb solution directly into the tumors at his center.

Cancer a Fungus problem?

Dr. Simonchini says that cancer is caused by fungus However, it is useful to know that not only does sodium bicarbonate disrupt the comfortable environment of tumors, but it also has anti-fungal effect.

Best Alternative Treatment - Budwig Protocol

90% documented success in all types of Cancers

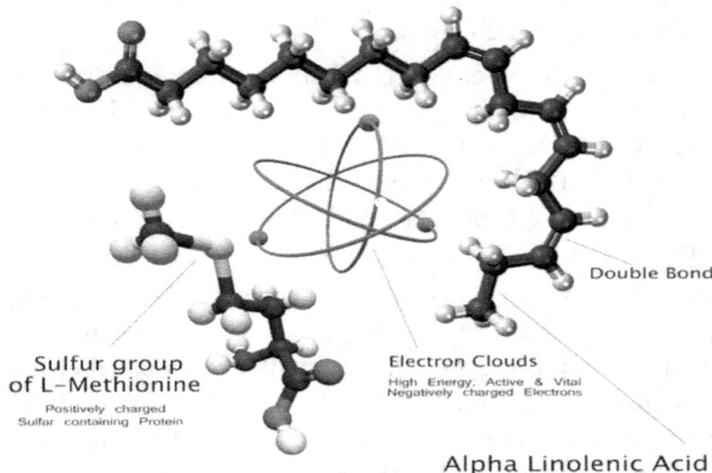

Dr. Budwig has been referred to as a top European cancer research scientist, biochemist, pharmacologist, and physicist. Dr. Budwig was a seven-time Nobel Prize nominee.

In Germany in 1952, she was the central government's senior expert for fats and pharmaceutical drugs. She's considered one of the world's leading authorities on fats and oils. Her research has shown the tremendous effects that commercially processed fats and oils (having Trans fatty acids) have in destroying cell membranes and lowering the voltage in the cells of our bodies, which then result in chronic and terminal disease including cancer.

What we have forgotten is that we are body electric. The cells of our body fire electrically. They have a nucleus in the center of the cell which is positively charged, and the cell membrane, which is the outer lining of the cell, is negatively charged. We are all aware of how fats clog up our veins and arteries and are the leading cause of heart attacks, but we never looked beyond the end of our noses to see how these very dangerous fats and oils are affecting the overall health of our minds and bodies at the cellular level.

Dr. Budwig discovered that when unsaturated fats have been chemically treated, their unsaturated qualities are destroyed and the field of electrons removed. This commercial processing of fats destroys the field of electrons that the cell membranes (60-75 trillion cells) in our bodies must have to fire properly (i.e. function properly).

The fats' ability to associate with protein and thereby to achieve water solubility in the fluids of the living body is destroyed. As Budwig put it, "the battery is dead because the electrons in these fats and oils recharge it." When the electrons are destroyed the fats are no longer active and cannot flow into the capillaries and through the fine capillary networks. This is when circulation problems arise.

Without the proper metabolism of fats in our bodies, every vital function and every organ is affected. This includes the generation of new life and new cells. Our bodies produce over 500 million new cells daily. Dr. Budwig points out that in growing new cells, there is a polarity between the electrically positive nucleus and the electrically negative cell membrane with its high unsaturated fatty acids. During cell division, the cell, and new daughter cell must contain enough electron-rich fatty acids in the cell's surface area to divide off completely from the old cell. When this process is interrupted the body begins to die. In essence, these commercially processed fats and oils are shutting down the electrical field of the cells allowing chronic and terminal diseases to take hold of our bodies.

A very good example would be tumors. Dr. Budwig noted that "The formation of tumors usually happens as follows. In those body areas which normally host many growth processes, such as in the skin and membranes, the glandular organs, for example, the liver and pancreas or the glands in the stomach and intestinal tract—it is here that the growth processes are brought to a standstill. Because the polarity is missing, due to the lack of electron rich highly unsaturated fat, the course of growth is disturbed—the surface-active fats are not present; the substance becomes inactive before the maturing and shedding process of the cells ever takes place, which results in the formation of tumors."

She pointed out that this can be reversed by providing the simple foods, cottage cheese, and flax seed oil, which revises the stagnated growth processes. This naturally causes the tumor or tumors present to dissolve and the whole range of symptoms which indicate a "dead battery are cured." Dr. Budwig did not believe in the use of growth-inhibiting treatments such as chemotherapy or radiation. She was quoted as saying "I flat declare that the usual hospital treatments today, in a case of tumorous growth, most certainly leads to worsening of the disease or a speedier death, and in healthy people, quickly causes cancer."

Dr. Budwig discovered that when she combined flaxseed oil, with its powerful healing nature of essential electron rich unsaturated fats, and cottage cheese, which is rich in sulfur protein, the bonding produced makes the oil water soluble and easily absorbed into the cell membrane.

I found testimonials of people from around the world who had been diagnosed with terminal cancer (all types of cancer), sent home to die and were now living healthy, normal lives. Not only had Dr. Budwig been using her protocol for treating cancer in Europe, but she also treated other chronic diseases such as arthritis, heart infarction, irregular heartbeat, psoriasis, eczema (other skin diseases), immune deficiency syndromes (Multiple Sclerosis and other autoimmune diseases), diabetes, lungs (respiratory conditions), stomach ulcers, liver, prostate, strokes, brain tumors, brain (strengthens activity), arteriosclerosis and other chronic diseases. Dr. Budwig's protocol proved successful where orthodox traditional medicine was failing.

Prime Cause of Cancer

We are fighting with cancer since the dawn of history. Every year we discover new diagnostic modalities, better radiotherapy techniques and lots of new chemotherapy drugs. But we have completely failed to defeat this disease called cancer. Think again, are we really going on the right path? Does conventional Medicine really targets upon the prime cause of cancer???

Otto Warburg – Biography

Otto Heinrich Warburg (October 8, 1883 – August 1, 1970), son of physicist Emil Warburg, was a German physiologist, medical doctor and Nobel laureate. His mother was the daughter of a Protestant family of bankers and civil servants from Baden. Warburg studied chemistry under the great Emil Fischer, and earned his "Doctor of Chemistry" in Berlin in 1906. He then earned the degree of "Doctor of Medicine" in Heidelberg in 1911. Between 1908 and 1914, Warburg was affiliated with the Naples Marine Biological Station, in Naples, Italy, where he conducted research.

He served as an officer in the elite Uhlan (cavalry regiment) during the First World War, and was given the Iron Cross (1st Class) award for his bravery. Warburg is considered one of the 20th century's leading biochemists. Towards the end of the war, Albert Einstein, who had been a friend of Warburg's father Emil, wrote Warburg asking him to leave the army and return to academia, since it would be a tragedy for the world to lose his talents. Einstein and Warburg later became friends, and Einstein's work in physics had great influence on Otto's biochemical research.

While working at the Marine Biological Station, Warburg performed research on oxygen consumption in sea urchin eggs after fertilization, and proved that upon fertilization, the rate of respiration increases by as much as six fold. His experiments also proved that iron is essential for the development of the larval stage.

In 1918, Warburg was appointed professor at the Kaiser Wilhelm Institute for Biology in Berlin-Dahlem. By 1931 he was promoted as director of the Kaiser Wilhelm Institute for Cell Physiology, which was later on, renamed the Max Planck Society. Warburg investigated the metabolism of tumors and the respiration of cells, particularly cancer cells, and in 1931 was awarded the Nobel Prize in Physiology for his "discovery of the nature and mode of action of the respiratory enzyme."

Nomination for a second Nobel Prize

In 1944, Warburg was nominated for a second Nobel Prize in Physiology by Albert Szent-Györgyi, for his work on nicotinamide, the mechanism and enzymes involved in fermentation, and the discovery of flavin (in yellow enzymes), but was prevented from receiving it by Adolf Hitler's regime.

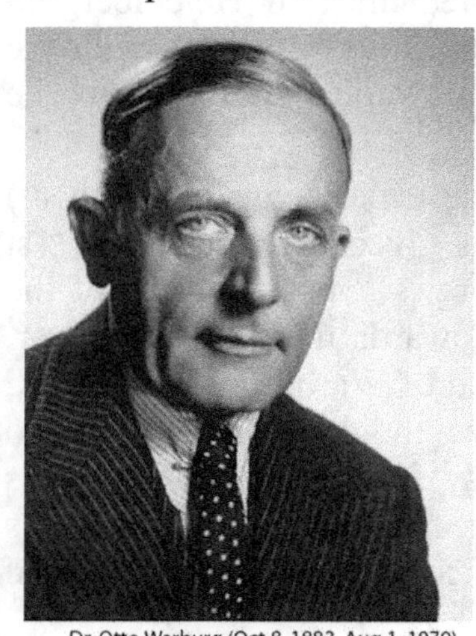
Dr. Otto Warburg (Oct 8, 1883 Aug 1, 1970)

Otto Warburg edited and had much of his original work published in The Metabolism of Tumors and wrote New Methods of Cell Physiology (1962). Otto Warburg was thrilled when Oxford University awarded him an honorary doctorate.

In his later years, Warburg was convinced that illness is resulted from pollution; this caused him to become a bit of a health advocate. He insisted on eating bread made from wheat grown organically on his farm. When he visited restaurants, he often made arrangements to pay the full price for a cup of tea, but to only be served boiling water, from which he would make tea with a tea bag he had brought with him. He was also known to go to significant lengths to obtain organic butter, the quality of which he trusted.

The Otto Warburg Medal

The Otto Warburg Medal is intended to commemorate Warburg's outstanding achievements. It has been awarded by the German Society for Biochemistry and Molecular Biology since 1963. The prize honors and encourages pioneering achievements in fundamental biochemical and molecular biological research. The Otto Warburg Medal is regarded as the highest award for biochemists and molecular biologists in Germany.

Prime cause of Cancer

Warburg hypothesized that cancer growth is caused by tumor cells mainly generating energy (as e.g. adenosine triphosphate / ATP) by anaerobic breakdown of glucose (known as fermentation, or anaerobic respiration). This is in contrast to healthy cells, which mainly generate energy from oxidative breakdown of pyruvate. Pyruvate is an end product of glycolysis, and is oxidized within the mitochondria. Hence, and according to Warburg, cancer should be interpreted as a mitochondrial dysfunction.

In short, Warburg summarized that all normal cells absolutely require oxygen, but cancer cells can live without oxygen - a rule without exception. Deprive a cell 35% of its oxygen for 48 hours and it would become cancerous. **Dr. Otto Warburg clearly mentioned that the root cause of cancer is lack of oxygen in the cells.**

He also discovered that cancer cells are anaerobic (do not breathe oxygen), get the energy by fermenting glucose and produce levo-rotating lactic acid, and the body becomes acidic. Cancer cannot survive in the presence of high levels of oxygen, as found in an alkaline state.

He postulated that sulfur containing protein and some unknown fat is required to attract oxygen into the cell. This fat plays a major role in the respiration and functioning of Warburg respiratory enzyme. He thought it would be butyric acid and made experiment, but this attempt was a failure. For many decades scientists were trying to identify this unknown and mysterious fat but nobody succeeded (Otto Warburg, Wikipedia).

Dr. Johanna Budwig - Biography & Science

Birth of an angel

A lovely couple, Hermann Budwig and Elisabeth, lived in Essen town of Germany situated on the bank of river Ruhr. On the eve of 30th September, 1908 Elisabeth delivered a brilliant and lucky angel. Hermann and 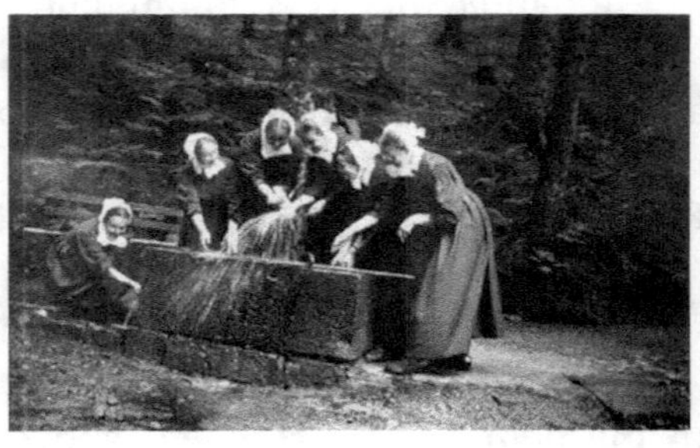 Elisabeth were very happy, and celebrating. They called her Johanna. In German, Johanna means a gift from God. In the family and neighborhood everybody was talking that Johanna is very lucky, she will study in a college and become a big doctor. Actually, 1908 was very fortunate and important year for the freedom of women in Germany. Government for the first time in history, changed laws, and allowed women to study in college and Universities. Also the German parliament passed a legislation to allow women to become members of political parties and prestigious clubs. Though women were given new rights and freedom, liberalization was slow and old values still persisted.

The tough life of a sage of science

Unluckily, Elisabeth died in 1920; family members thought that her father, being a poor loco mechanic, might not look after Johanna. So she was sent to an orphanage. This was a great shock for the little Johanna, but it had one positive side also. Education up to higher level was totally free for orphans.

In 1926, Germany was slowly recovering from the after effects of the First World War. Economic conditions were improving. Scholars and scientists were developing new technologies in every field. One third of all Nobel Prizes were being given to German academics.

Deaconess at Kaiserswerth

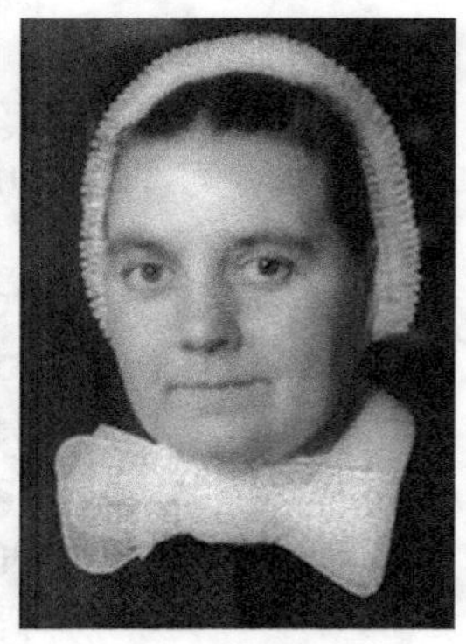

Johanna was very intelligent and sharp in studies from the beginning. In order to achieve good future, she decided to join the renowned Deaconess's Institute of Kaiserswerth in 1925. Theodor Fliedner, a pastor, founded Kaiserswerth Institute for welfare of unmarried mothers, prisoners, patients, orphans and poor children in 1836. In the beginning a Hospital and a Nursing School was established. This school was very famous Nursing School of that time. Florence Nightingale, known as mother of modern nursing, also studied in this Deaconess School in 1850. Intelligent Johanna easily got admission in this Institute. She was made a "deaconess" on March 30, 1932. This was the most appropriate place for her. There was a 1000 bedded hospital, pharmacy and a boarding school. She decided to study pharmacy.

After completing preliminary education in Kaiserswerth, she joined Münster University for further studies. Her analytical thinking and precise knowledge was noticed by her Professor Dr Hans Paul Kaufmann. He always encouraged and helped her. Here she passed state examination in pharmacy and was rewarded distinction in chemistry in 1936. Then she continued further education in physics, and received the title "Doctor of Science" at the University of Münster in 1938. On August 1, 1939, she was appointed as in-charge of pharmacy at the Military Hospital in Kaiserswerth.

Next month, Hitler's military forces attacked Poland. During war time, brave Johanna was busy in organizing and expanding the pharmacy. The war was not an easy time. There were two thousand people living in Kaiserswerth. Johanna was responsible for ensuring that there were enough medicines in this time of rationing and a thriving black market. She was well prepared and ready to fulfill any emergency demand for her patients. Many of her fellow deaconesses were often jealous and not co-operating but she continued evolving her professional skills. She was strong and was confronting every opponent (Dr. Johanna Budwig Stiftung).

Dr Budwig's scientific thinking, work and career

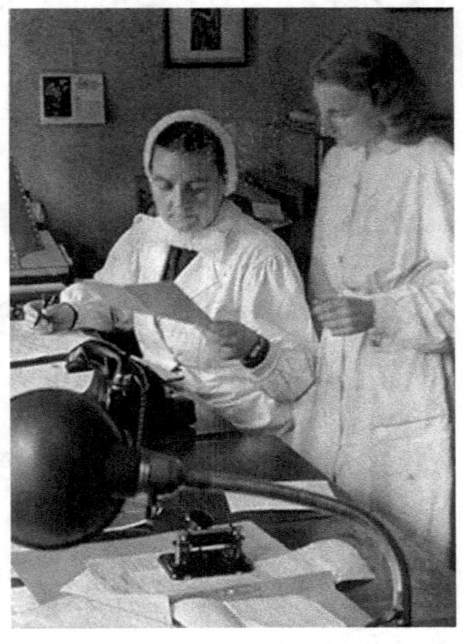

After Second World War, Johanna left Kaiserswerth in 1949. Soon Prof. Kaufmann came to know that she had left Kaiserswerth. He immediately met and persuaded her to work with him in Münster University, as he was always impressed from her talent. He converted the basement of his house into a laboratory and arranged all facilities for her research. He was famous as Fat Pope in the whole Europe.

On Prof. Kaufmann's recommendation, Johanna was appointed as the chief expert for drugs and fats at the Federal Institute for Fats Research, Germany. This was the country's largest office issuing the approval of new drugs used for cancer. Many applications had been submitted to her for approval. These were the medications for cancer therapy with the sulfhydryl group (sulfur-containing protein compounds). Everywhere she saw that fats played a role in cellular respiration, also in expert reports provided by well-known professors like Prof. Nonnenbruch. Unfortunately, fats could only be detected in the late stage, and there were no method to distinguish between fats chemically.

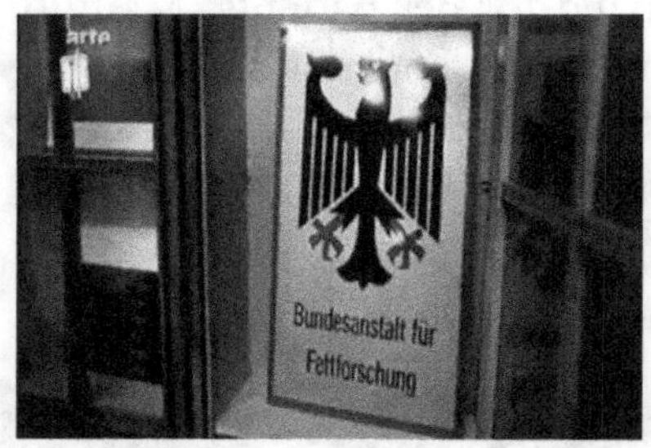

By this time, she developed paper chromatography. With this technique for first time she was able to detect fatty acids and lipoproteins directly even in 0.1 ml of blood. She used Co60 isotopes successfully to produce the first differential reaction for fatty acids, and produced the first direct iodine value via radioiodine. She also developed control of atmosphere in a closed system by using gas systems which act as antioxidants. She further developed Coloring methods, separating effects of fats and fatty acids. She too studied their behavior in blue and red light with fluorescent dyes.

Using rhodamine red dye, she studied the electrical behavior of the unsaturated fatty acids with their "halo". With this technique she could prove that electron rich highly unsaturated Linoleic and Linolenic fatty acids (Flax oil being the richest source) were the mysterious and undiscovered decisive fats required to attract oxygen into the cells, which Otto Warburg could not find. She studied the electromagnetic function of pi-electrons of the linolenic acid in the cell membranes, for nerve function, secretions, mitosis, as well as cell division. She also examined the synergism of the sulfur containing protein with the

pi-electrons of the highly unsaturated fatty acids and their significance for the formation of the hydrogen bridge between fat and protein, which represent "the only path" for fast and focused Transport of electrons during respiration. This research was extensively

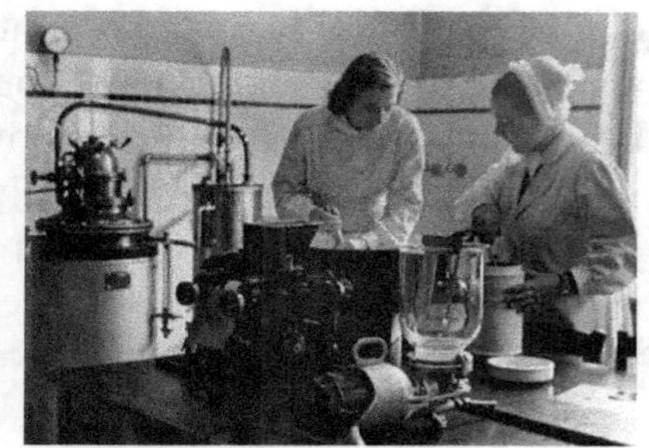

published in 1950 in Neue Wege in der Fettforschung (New Directions in Fat Research) and other publications.

This immediately caused an excitement and turmoil in the scientific community. Everybody thought that it would open new doors in Cancer research. She also proved that hydrogenated fats and refined oils including all Trans-fatty acids were not having vital electrons and were respiratory poisons.

During her research, she found that the blood of seriously ill cancer patients had deficiency of unsaturated essential fats (Linoleic and Linolenic fatty acids), lipoproteins, phosphatides, and hemoglobin. She also had noticed that cancer 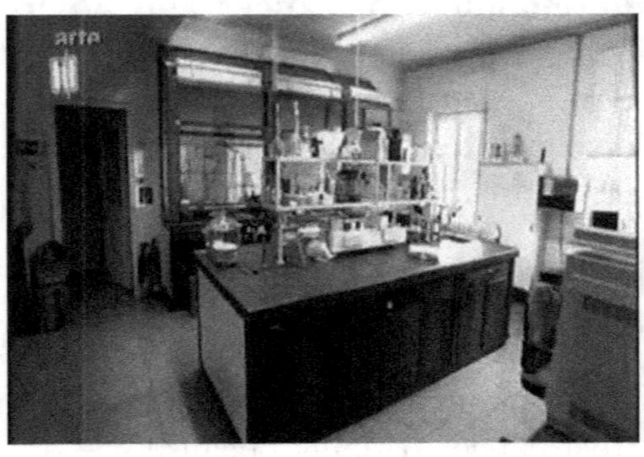 patients had a strange greenish-yellow substance in their blood which is not present in the blood of healthy people (Budwig, Cancer The Problem And The Solution).

She wanted to develop a healing program for cancer. So she enrolled over 642 cancer patients from four hospitals in Münster. She gave Flax oil and Cottage Cheeseto these patients. After just three months, patients began to improve in health and strength, the yellow green substance in their blood began to disappear, tumors gradually receded and at the same time the nutrients began to rise.

This way she developed a simple cure for cancer, based on the consumption of Flax oil with low fat Quark or cottage cheese, raw organic diet, mild exercise, Flax oil massage and the healing powers of the sun. It was a great victory and the first milestone in the battle against cancer. She treated approx. 2500 cancer patients during last few decades. Prof. Halme of surgery clinic in Helsinki used to keep records of her patients. According to him her success was over 90%, and this was achieved in cases, which were rejected by Allopathic doctors.

Dr. Budwig was a courageous scientist. She **loudly and convincingly argued that consumption of highly processed foods, particularly edible oils and margarines, which block the oxidation processes in the cells, are responsible for the development of cancer and other degenerative diseases.** She met with great resistance from food industry giants, who were doing everything to prevent the spread of her sensational discovery. In 1952, under the influence of strong pressure from this lobby, she lost her job and was barred from the research work.

Joins Medical School at Göttingen

Opponents of Dr. Johanna blamed her that she should not treat cancer patients because she doesn't have a doctor's degree. She felt this and eventually joined medical school in Göttingen in

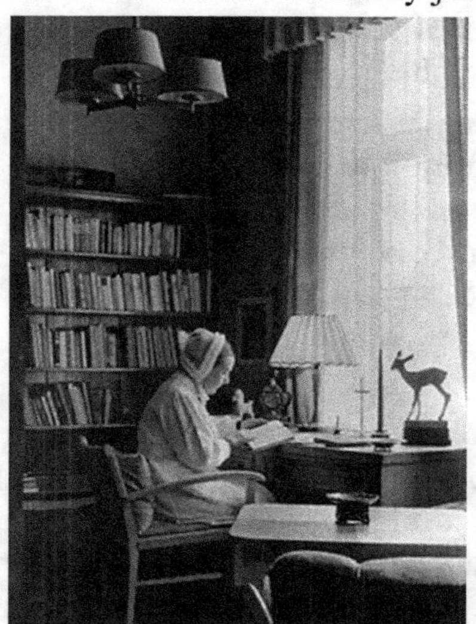

1955. Budwig was 47 years old at that time. She also continued her research work along with her studies. *Budwig successfully treated Prof. Martius's wife, who suffered from Breast Cancer*

One night a woman came with her small child whose arm was supposed to be amputated due to a tumor. She treated her and soon the amputation surgery was dismissed, and the child quickly did very well.

A Swiss woman came to her clinic in Göttingen. She suffered from Colon Cancer with metastasis and intestinal obstruction. Several doctors examined her, and were to be operated on Christmas Eve. On Budwig's request, she was treated by her protocol. The tumor of the colon quickly subsided. Seven weeks later, she was discharged without any detectable tumor. It is interesting that the Swiss custom officer was not ready to believe that the submitted passport belonged to same lady. Her look was so much changed! At home her daughter welcomed saying: "You look healthy, younger and more beautiful (from her book The Death of the Tumor – Vol. II).

After this, University allowed her to treat cancer patients with her oil-protein diet. She was getting miraculous results. University professors were excited with the results, but wanted that she should also include chemo and radiotherapy. She was rigid and didn't want to compromise. So she had differences and conflicts with her professors and ultimately left Göttingen (Budwig, Cancer The Problem And The Solution).

Last Destination - Dietersweiler-Freudenstadt

Eventually, she shifted to Dietersweiler-Freudenstadt, where she lived till her death. There she completed Ph.D. in Naturopathy so that she could legally treat cancer patients. She continued treating her patients in Freudenstadt. In 1968 she created unique Eldi oils for massage and enema, called Electron Differential Oils after performing precise spectroscopic measurements of the light absorption in different oils. *US pain institute has written somewhere: "What this crazy woman does with her ELDI oils, none of us manages to do via pain killers."*

Budwig conducted more than 200 lectures worldwide. Dr. Budwig was popular in the U.S. as FLAX SEED lady from Freudenstadt. She delivered her last public Lecture in Freudenstadt on March 3, 1999. On November 28, 2002, she fell down in her bathroom and got a fracture in right femur neck. She was admitted in a nursing home and ultimately died on May 19, 2003.

Budwig Protocol

The Budwig Protocol is one of the most widely followed alternative treatments for cancer and other diseases. The diet seems simple, but foods are powerful and can heal a person.

Transition Diet

The Transition diet is especially recommended for patients of liver, pancreatic or gall bladder cancers. The basic principle is that for 3 days nothing is eaten and drunk except the following written and at least three times daily warm tea (herbal teas from peppermint, rose hip, mallow or green tea) is drunk. Dr Budwig has recommended variant 1 for patients with a relatively good energy state, and variant 2 and 3 mainly for seriously ill patients.

Variant 1

Variant 1 for three days, 250 g of linomel or alternatively freshly crushed Flax seed is eaten together with the following:

- Freshly pressed fruit juices without added sugar.
- Freshly pressed vegetable juices such as carrot, celery juice, red beetroots and apple juice.
- Chinese tea and black tea are allowed in the morning
- Honey for sweetening is allowed. Just as grape juice for drinking and as a sweetener. Energetically weak patients can also consume sparkling wine and linomel.

Variant 2

For three days, oat meal cereal very hour with linomel is eaten daily with the following juices:

- Freshly pressed fruit juices or freshly pressed vegetable juices such as carrot, celery juice, beetroot and apple juice.
- Chinese tea and black tea are allowed in the morning.
- Honey for sweetening is allowed. Just as grape juice for drinking and as a sweetener.

- Energetically weak patients can also consume sparkling wine and linomel.

Variant 3

For three days, oatmeal soup with linomel is given three times a day together with the following juices:

- Freshly pressed fruit juices or fruit juices without added sugar.
- Freshly pressed vegetable juices such as carrot, celery juice, beetroot and apple juice.
- Chinese tea and black tea are allowed in the morning.
- Honey for sweetening is allowed. Just as grape juice for drinking and as a sweetener.
- Energetically weak patients can also consume sparkling wine and linomel.

It is often experienced frequently that patients mixed all three variants and "nevertheless" had good results. So better you to stick to one variant. (Budwig – Cancer The Problem And The Solution 2005: p.36).

Budwig Diet

The Budwig Protocol is necessary for many diseases from cancer to type 2 diabetes and heart disease to autoimmune diseases, etc. Its purpose is to energize the cells by restoring the natural electrical potential in the cell. Many human diseases are caused by "sick cells" which have lost their normal electrical potential; generally via a lower ATP energy in the cell's mitochondria.

6:00 AM – Sauerkraut juice

A glass of sauerkraut juice consumed before breakfast every morning. It is rich in vitamins including C, enzymes and helps develop the health-promoting gut flora. Sauerkraut is cabbage that has been pickled by natural fermentation, mainly with lactobacillus bacteria. It is slightly salty, sharp and sour. Well made, it is much nicer than it sounds. You may also consume another glass of sauerkraut juice later in the day.

It interesting that sauerkraut contains right rotating lactic acids and is highly alkaline and neutralizes levo-rotating lactic acids and makes our body alkaline. That is why Marcus Porcius Cato the Elder issued a statement - Carcinomas are incurable except with the treatment with Sauerkraut.

8:00 AM Breakfast

Green or herbal tea

Start breakfast with a cup of warm herbal or green tea. Sweeten with only natural honey. You can add lemon or grape juice. Patient should take such a tea before or with Linomel Muesli. You may consume 4-5 such teas in a day.

Linomel Muesli or Oil-Protein Muesli

This should be made fresh and consumed within 15 minutes.

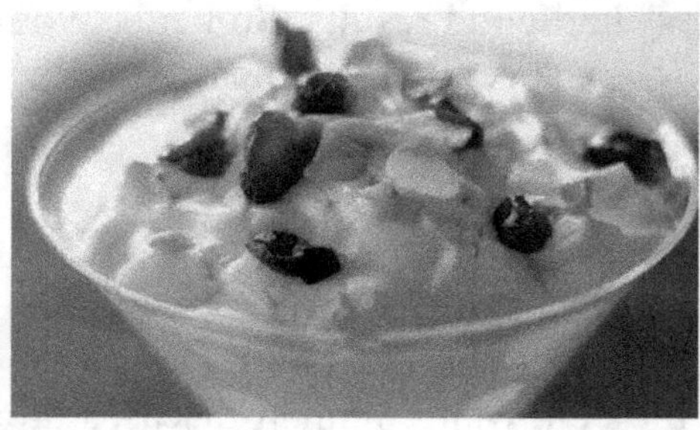

It is full of high energy pi-electrons, attract oxygen in the cells and capable of healing cell membranes. It is full of energy-rich omega-3 fats, has power to attract healing photons from sun through resonance. As "Om" is divine word and synonym of God in India. According to Hindu Mythology, the whole universe is located inside "Om", so the name Omkhand has been given to this wonderful recipe in Hindi.

Ingredients

- 3 Tbsp cold pressed organic Flax seed oil (FO)
- 100-125gm (6 Tbsp) Quark or Cottage Cheese(CC)
- 2 Tbsp freshly ground Flax seeds
- 2 Tbsp milk
- 1 cup fruits
- ¼ cup dried nuts

- Natural honey
- Flavorings – lemon, apple cider vinegar, cinnamon, pure cacao, natural vanilla, shredded coconut etc.

Recipe

Place 2 tablespoons Linomel or freshly ground Flax seeds in a small bowl. It is covered with raw, crushed or diced seasonal fruits depending on the season. Pour some orange or grape juice over this. Linomel^{Tm} is a brand name and originally created and patented by Budwig. It is a cereal made from cracked Flax Seed, a small amount of honey and a little milk powder.

Then the Quark-Flax seed oil cream is prepared in as follows: First add Flax seed oil, milk and honey and blend briefly with a hand-held immersion electric blender, then gradually add the Quark in smaller portions. Blend till oil and Quark is thoroughly mixed with no separated oil. Then it is seasoned differently everyday with different flavorings such as vanilla, cinnamon or various fruits such as banana, apple, lemon, orange juice, or berries.

Use various fruits such as fresh berries, apple, cherry, orange, banana, papaya, grapes etc. Add other fresh fruit if you like, totaling ½ to 1 cup of fruit. Budwig specially advised to use berries like strawberry, blueberry, raspberry, cheery

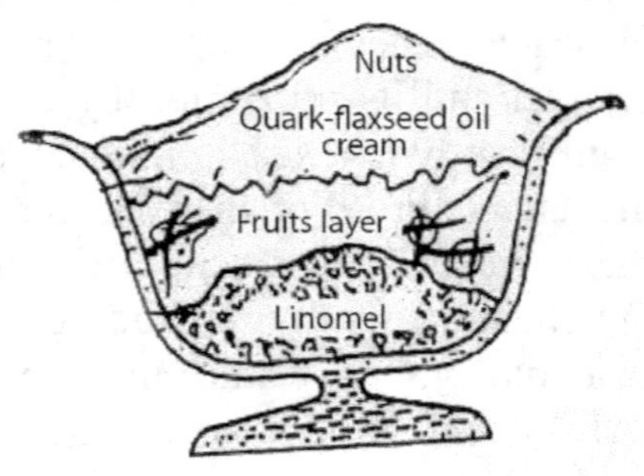

etc. because berries have ellagic acids which are strong cancer fighters.

Add organic raw nuts such as walnuts, almonds, raisins or Brazil nuts. They have sulfurated proteins, omega-3 fats and vitamins. Brazil nut is especially important because a single nut provides you with all of the selenium you need for the day.

Selenium is very important to boost immune power. Peanuts are prohibited.

For variety and flavor, try natural vanilla, cinnamon, lemon juice, pure cocoa or shredded coconut.

Once blended in Budwig Cream, Quark and Flax seed oil form a new substance called lipoprotein. Lipoprotein is a water soluble complex. The Quark is rich in the sulfur-containing amino acids, methionine and cysteine. These positively charged amino acids attract the negatively charged electron clouds in fatty acid chains and exhibit a stabilizing effect on the highly unsaturated, otherwise easily oxidized fats. Thus, the amino acids protect the polyunsaturated fatty acids from the Flax seed oil against oxidation which, as a result, are able to enter the human body unchanged and with their full energy potential. The result: they are much more valuable to cells and their membranes. Consequently, one could say that Quark excels as a protector for the polyunsaturated fatty acids.

Sulfur-rich amino acids play a wealth of roles in many vital functions in our bodies. In combination with polyunsaturated fatty acids, they are important partners in regulating the uptake of oxygen and its utilization by the cell. They therefore contribute significantly to a strong immune system, healthy metabolism, and mental vitality. For many generations, people have been getting their omega-3 fatty acids from fish, vegetables, nuts, and seeds. Our health literally depends on the regular consumption of the essential omega-3 and omega-6 fatty acids, alpha-linolenic acid (ALA) and linoleic acid (LA). Our bodies require these fatty acids in order to synthesize their cell membranes as well as for a variety of metabolic processes and heal the cancer and other diseases.

Tips for making the Budwig Mixture

- Follow directions properly! It is important to add things to the mixture in the right order. If you mix them in the wrong order you may lose a lot of the opportunity to convert the oil-soluble omega-3 into water soluble-omega-3.
- Keep the Flax seed oil refrigerated.
- Immersion blender is a must.
- The mixture can be flavored differently every day by adding nuts and fruits preferably organic such as pecans, almonds or walnuts (not peanuts), banana, organic cocoa, shredded coconut, pineapple (fresh) blueberries, raspberries, cinnamon, vanilla or (freshly) squeezed fruit juice.
- Consume immediately for best results.

10 AM Vegetable juice

Freshly squeezed vegetable juice from carrots, beets, celery, tomato, and radish, lemon as well as green vegetables - stinging nettle, lettuce or spinach. Apple is added to sweeten and enhance the taste. Carrot & beet juices are especially helpful to the liver and have strong cancer fighting properties. Vary vegetables. Some tasty and nutritious combinations are beet and apple juice, carrot and apple, carrot and beet, asparagus and apple, celery and apple, celery and carrot. Beet juice should not be taken alone. If taken alone it may cause red or pink urine (beeturia).

She also frequently recommended the following juices:

1. Nettle juice - Especially in the spring, Dr Budwig recommended to puree nettles with water and a lemon.

2. Radish juice - For this, a radish is first crushed and then thrown together with a lemon into the juicer. This juice is by the way durable for several days and Dr Budwig has sometimes recommended her patients to drink a small quantity of them every day.

3. Coltsfoot juice - For this juice, with the exception of the harder old rootstock, the entire remaining underground shoot is mixed with a few flowers and some milk and honey.

4. Horseradish juice - Mix 3-5 cm horseradish together with an apple and (raw) milk. Depending on the quantity of milk you can change the taste. Dr Budwig recommended this juice above all to workmen and to stimulate the appetite. Freshly pressed means, by the way, that you drink the juice within 5 minutes after pressing. In some cases, Dr Budwig prescribed a second juice 30 to 60 minutes later.

12:15 PM Lunch

Salad Platter: Salad plate with homemade cottage cheese-Flax seed mayonnaise. As salad also use: dandelion, cress, celery, tomato, cucumber, lettuce, radish, cabbage, broccoli, green horseradish and pepper.

Delicious mayo salad dressing can be prepared by mixing together 2 Tbsp (30 ml) Flax Oil, 2 Tbsp (30 ml) milk, and 2 Tbsp (30 ml) cottage cheese. Then add 2 tablespoons (30 ml) of Lemon juice (or Apple Cider Vinegar) and add 1 teaspoon (2.5 g) Mustard powder plus some herbs of your choice. Other alternative dressing can be made by mixing Flax Oil, lemon juice, Mustard and some herbs (Budwig, The Oil-Protein Diet Cookbook, 1994).

Main Course: Vegetables cooked in water, then flavored with Oleolox and herbs possibly with oatmeal, soy sauce, curry etc. Vegetable broth flavored with

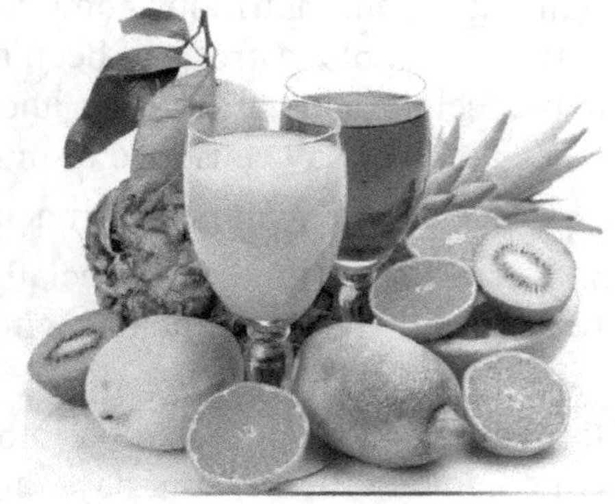

a little Oleolox and yeast flakes. As side dish for the vegetables: buckwheat, brown rice, millet or potatoes can be used. One or two slices of Ezekiel bread can be taken. Use lot of dried fruits in the main meal also.

Lunch Dessert: Cottage cheese/ Flax oil mixture served as a dessert, prepared with dry fruits and fruits such as apple, or poured over a fruit salad. You already know how to prepare it perfectly. You will find wonderful recipes for a delicious dessert in the Oil-Protein cookbook by Budwig. Please note that the dessert is **"a must"** and should definitely be eaten. So keep your main course light so you may enjoy the dessert happily.

The form of preparation as "fruit foam," "Linovita" or "red coat in the snow" (in Oil-Protein cookbook) is always welcoming for the healthy and the sick. In all the gimmicks in the preparation of the delicious desserts, one should be aware: Quark and Flaxseed give the patient immense power within a short space of time. Always fresh and beautiful, always freshly interesting, this important food for life should be for the sick and for the whole family.

3 PM Fruit juices

In the afternoon, Dr Budwig recommended different kinds of fruit juices e.g. apples, grapes, cherries, pineapples, papaya, or apricot, sparkling wine or wine - with or without Flaxseeds or with or without a few drops Flaxseed oil.

Budwig preferred papaya juice and recommended her patients to drink at least every 2 days a glass of papaya juice. The main reason for this was definitely the protein splitting enzyme papain.

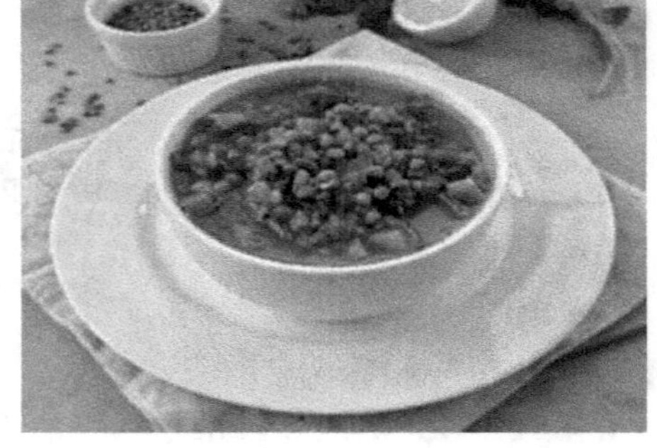

6 PM Dinner

The evening meal should be light and served early, around 6 p.m. A warm meal may be prepared using brown rice, buckwheat or oat meal. Never consume corn or soy beans. Dishes made with buckwheat grouts are most easily tolerated and nourishing. Use only honey to sweeten. Soup or more solid dishes can be combined with a tasty sauce according to preference. Use OLEOLOX liberally also to sweet sauces and soups, making them nourishing and a richer source of energy.

8:30 PM

A glass of organic red wine may be consumed. All things are a matter of correct dosage. This glass of red wine is not a "must" program. In fact, seriously ill patients having pain and discomfort just starting on the oil-protein diet, it is recommended to serve a glass of red wine mixed with freshly ground Flax seeds to tide them over while going off pain killers (Budwig, Cancer The Problem And The Solution).

METRIC CONVERSION TABLE	
10 g = 0.35 oz	5 cc = 1 teaspoon
100 g = 3.5 oz	15 cc = 1 tablespoon
150 g = 5.25 oz	30 cc = 1 ounce
250 g = 8.8 oz	250 cc = 1 cup
454 g = 1 lb	960 cc = 1 qt
Oz = ounce lb = pound qt = quart Tsp = teaspoon Tbsp = tablespoon	

Precautions

Drink filtered water - Use RO (Reverse Osmosis)water for drinking, cooking and enemas.

Eat Organic Diet - Always try to eat organic food.

Dental Care –

Mercury is a Carcinogenic as well as a Poison! The root canals of dead teeth are full of bacteria that attack the liver and lymphatic system. From Amalgam fillings the mercury slowly leaks out of the filings. The ADA cleverly defends the use of amalgam in spite of the fact that there is sufficient evidence that patients with many severe problems, including psychotic episodes and fatal allergic reactions, were just cured by removing the amalgam. It is advisable to rather have a ceramic filling than be slowly poisoned by mercury. Even gold filling is dangerous; it acts as battery producing electrical current. Be informed that the effect of drugs, including poison, is dose dependant and cumulative.

Fluoride is not only toxic but it is also carcinogenic. Fluoride has never been proven to prevent tooth decay. It has been outlawed in many countries or groups of countries because the evidence is overwhelming that fluoride causes premature aging, so drink bottled water and use fluoride-free toothpaste (American Cancer Institute - 1963).

I highly recommend helping you avoid fillings in the first place. Holistic dentist recommend 3% H_2O_2 as a gargle or rinse, or making a paste using baking soda. H_2O_2 usage three times a day is advised. It is great for cleaning dentures, too.

Frying and deep frying - Frying and deep frying is not allowed to cook patient's food. Never heat any oil in the kitchen. By heating oils the wealth of high energy electrons is destroyed and Trans fats and dangerous toxic chemicals such as acrylamides are formed in the oil. Boiling and steaming are good practices. You can fry vegetables etc. in water and add oleolox before

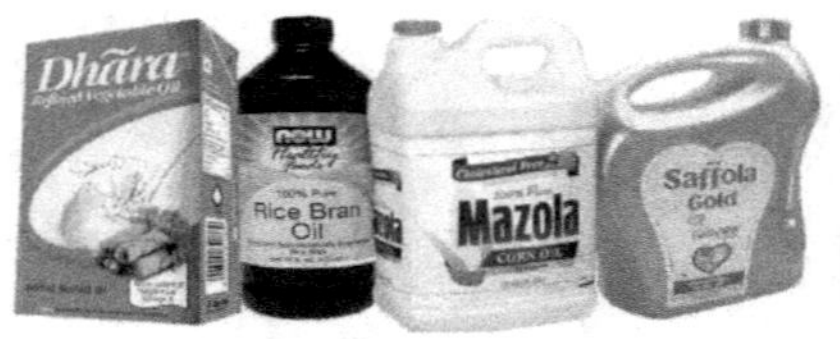

serving. Water is the safest medium for frying, says Lothar Hirneise.

Chemo and Radio -

Chemotherapy is aimed at destruction of the tumor, and it destroys many living cells, and the entire person. Anything that disturbs growth is fatal because growth is an elementary 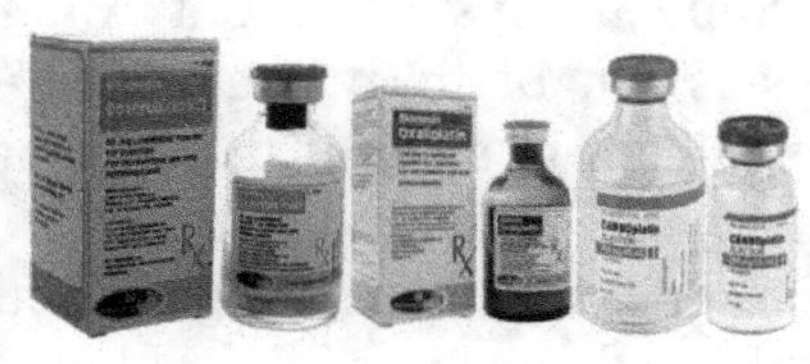 function of life. We cannot achieve something good with bad tools.

Dr. Budwig rejects Chemo and Radiation Therapy. Budwig used to say with full confidence and clarity, "My treatment targets on the real cause of cancer; it fills cancer cells with high energy pi-electrons and attracts oxygen into the cells. And cancer cells start to breathe and produce vital energy."

Man-made Supplements - With this treatment man-made antioxidants, synthetic vitamins and pain killers should not be given. The dose of anticoagulants and aspirin should be adjusted by your doctor. Dr. Budwig favors natural, herbal and homeopathy instead of man-made and synthetic supplements, vitamins and pain killers (Budwig, Cancer The Problem And The Solution).

Prohibitions of Budwig Protocol

In this protocol there are certain restrictions. They are as important as the diet itself. It is very difficult to defeat the cancer without strictly following these rules.

Sugar is strictly forbidden

Sugar, Jiggery, molasses, maple syrup and artificial sweeteners like xylitol, aspartame are not permitted. You can use only natural honey, stevia and fruit juices – all off course unprocessed.

Avoid meats, eggs and fish

Meat, fish, poultry, eggs, and butter are never allowed. Preserved meat is like a poison. It is highly processed and treated with dangerous antibiotics, preservatives and nitrates.

Stop using Hydrogenated Fat and Refined oil

You can never eat pizza, burger, fast food, fried food, biscuits etc. as they all are made by hydrogenated margarine and shortenings. Hydrogenation is a very dangerous process, used to increase shelf life of fats. In this process (oil is heated at very high temperature and hydrogen is passed through oils in presence of nickel) killing Trans fats are formed, high energy live and vital electrons are destroyed and nutrients are damaged. Hydrogenated Fats is just a dead, nutrition-less and cancer causing liquid plastic. Budwig always preached against these damaging fats. She has allowed low fat cheese, oleolox and coconut oil.

Preservatives and Processed Food

You should not eat Potato chips, soft drinks etc. which are full of preservatives. Never consume highly processed food e.g. ready to eat packed foods, pasta, pastries, bread and soy products, tofu etc. However good quality soy souse is permitted.'

Microwave, Teflon, Aluminum and Plastic

Never cook in microwave oven. Food cooked in microwave become toxic and deformed. Also don't use aluminum, plastic, Teflon coated cookware and aluminum foils. Use stainless steel, iron, china clay or glass utensils instead.

Chemicals and pesticides are not allowed

Avoid pesticides and chemicals, even those in household products & cosmetics. Stay away from mosquito repellants, sun screen lotions and sun glasses.

Wear natural fibers

Don't wear clothes made using synthetic fiber like nylon, polyester and acrylic. Budwig put great emphasis on the fact that her patients only wore natural fabrics such as cotton or satin, since they too can influence the magnetic field of our body.

Bed

Don't use on foam pillow and mattress. She recommended horsehair mattresses. Latex mattresses are the second choice. In any case, however, you should always replace mattresses that have metal spring cores.

CRT TV and mobile phones

These emit dangerous electromagnetic radiation, so do not use them. You can watch LCD and plasma TVs.

No left over

Food should be prepared fresh and eaten soon after preparation to maximize intake of health giving electrons and enzymes (Budwig, Cancer The Problem And The Solution).

Few Desserts recipes by Dr. Budwig

Fujiya delight

Ingredients for 3 people:

250 cc grape juice, 250 cc pure currant juice,
8g agar-agar, Quark-Flaxseed oil,
Milk, honey, vanilla cream

Preparation:

Heat the grape juice till it boils, then add the currant juice, agar-agar, stirring constantly for 5 minutes, and allow to cool. Now divide this mass to 3 narrow, tall cups, which have been rinsed with cold water. It is preferable if these cups have a bottom diameter of only 3- 4 cm. Refrigerate to cool. Now mix a Quark-Flaxseed oil cream with milk, honey and vanilla. Turn the red jelly upside down onto glass plates. The Quark-Flaxseed oil cream is placed on the top so that only the upper half is covered with the Quark-Flaxseed oil cream, so that top looks like the Snow caped Mount Fujiyama.

(The beautiful hotel with a gorgeous view of the Fujiyama is called "Fujiya", hence the dessert "Fujiya".)

Linovita-in-love in wine jelly

Ingredients: for 5 people:

250 cc of grape juice, 250 ccm of white wine,
8 agar-agar, 4 tablespoons of milk,
8 tablespoons of Flaxseed oil, 2 teaspoons of honey,
200-250 g of Quark, 2 liqueur glasses
Vodka, plum (Slibowitz) or cherry brandy or rum

Preparation:

The wine jelly is prepared by heating 250 cc of grape juice till it boils. Agar-agar is stirred with a little wine and placed in the boiling grape juice. Immediately remove from the cooking plate and add the remaining wine gradually with constant stirring. After about 5 minutes, the jelly mixture clears itself. You can now divide to approx. 5 glass bowls or champagne glasses. Immediately afterwards, mix the Quark-Flaxseed oil cream from Flaxseed oil, milk, honey and Quark. Finally, add 2 liqueur glasses of vodka or slibovitz or cherry brandy or rum into the Quark-Flaxseed oil cream. This Quark-Flaxseed oil mixture is evenly divided on the ready to-use bowls so that the Quark-Flaxseed oil cream partly sinks down in the middle. It is served after complete solidification.

Ice cream with cocoa

Ingredients:

3 tablespoons of Flaxseed oil, 3 tablespoons of milk,
1 tablespoon of honey, 100g of Quark, 100 g of hazelnuts,
2 tablespoons of cocoa

Preparation:

Quark, Flaxseed oil, milk and honey are mixed in the blender, then the hazelnuts are added, well blended and finally, cocoa is added to the mixture. Now pour the entire mixture into the ice-maker and place it in the fridge compartment of the refrigerator. This mixture with a nougat flavor gives the various combinations mentioned here the dark color contrasts. For very ill people these preparations are very important, especially when there is a general lack of appetite.

(Oil-Protein Diet by Lothar Hirneise available at http://www.hirneise.com/page-8/page-19/)

ELDI oils

Dr. Budwig created unique ELDI oils, called electron differential oils after performing precise spectroscopic measurements of the light absorption in different oils - specifying that the oils contained pi-electron clouds from Flax oil, wheat germ oil plus vitamin-E in its natural complex, etheric oils and sulfhydryl groups.

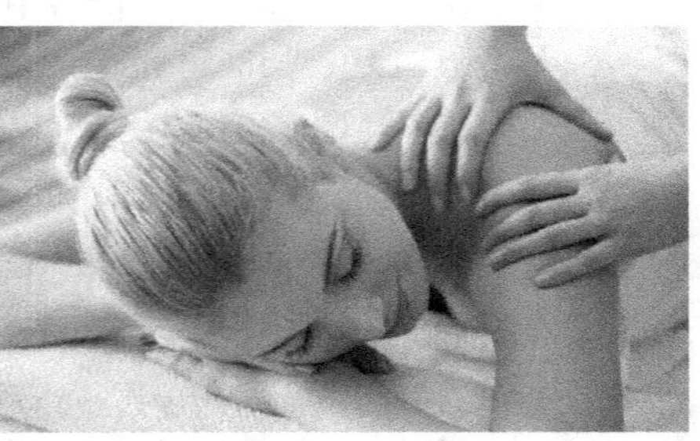

Dr. Johanna Budwig said, "The sun is my preferred treatment modality, as is ELDI oil, used externally to stimulate the absorption of the long-wave band of the sun. I have used ELDI oils extensively since 1968 for body massage as well as in the selective application of oil packs. US pain institute has written somewhere: "What this crazy woman does with her ELDI oils, none of us manages to do via pain killers." Dr. Budwig has mentioned that if ELDI oil is not available, you may use Flax oil instead. *You can buy ELDI oils at: www.sensei.de*

Massage Benefits

- Since ancient time massage has been part of cancer healing. Think of your lymphatics as a trash-disposal system for your body. Massage initiates lymphatic drainage, you push the trash out of your body and you're helping your immune system.
- Massage therapy is sometimes the first really pleasant touch a patient is able to experience.
- Massage also releases endorphins (our body's natural painkillers), stimulates lymph movement, and stretches tissues throughout the body. It's energizing, stimulating, and pretty good feeling.

ELDI oil plans:

A: For cancer patients in support of the energy level
1. Full-body rubbings in the morning
2. ELDI oil R enema with 200ml every 2-3 days
3. Wrap at the "place of the happening"

B: For energetically weak patients
1. Full-body rubbings in the morning and in the evening
2. Enema: standard plan for ELDI oil R
3. Wrap at the "place of the happening"
4. Daily liver wrap with ELDI oil sage

Additional information:

- Make sure that you make once a week an (deep/high) enema with water or coffee.
- If you make daily coffee enemas, then start in the morning with the coffee enema and then with the ELDI R enema, but only if your energetic level allows you to make two enemas daily. Otherwise, only make the ELDI R enema. (Oil Protein Diet by Lothar Hirneise)

ELDI oils from SENSEI (www.sensei.de) are produced in a permanent cold chain in a European oil mill and marketed under the name of Electron Differentiation Oils. There are two qualities. A 6-star organic quality and a 5-star quality, which are produced exclusively for the IOPDF (www.iopdf.com).

Cost factor ELDI oils

Again and again we hear that for reasons of cost, patients use Flax seed oil instead of ELDI oil R for an enema. Please do not do so, because Flax seed oil does not react in the same way as ELDI oil R. Instead, use cheap ELDI oils from IOPDF or reduce the amount of oil.

Procedure –

Two times a day, i.e. morning and evening, rub ELDI Oil or Flax oil into the skin over the whole body, a bit more intensely on the shoulders, armpits and groin area (where plenty of lymphatic vessels are present) as well as the problem areas, such as the breast, stomach, liver, etc. Leave the oil on the skin for about 20 minutes and follow with a warm water shower without washing with soap. After 10 minutes take another shower, this time using a mild soap, and then relax for 15-20 minutes.

Once the body has been oiled and the ELDI Oil or Flax oil has penetrated the skin, the warm water will open the skin pores and the oil penetrates the skin more deeply. The second shower, where one washes with soap, cleanses the skin so that clothes and linen will not become overly soiled.

Oil Packs

Take a piece of cloth made of pure cotton. Cut to a size to fit the body part, such as the knee. Soak the cotton cloth with oil, place on the knee etc., cover it with a piece of polythene and wrap it up with an elastic bandage. Leave overnight. Remove in the morning and wash the knee; repeat in the evening. Keep applying the same procedure for weeks, you get good results. You also use Flax oil or castor oil for these local applications if you do not get ELDI oils . Dr Budwig generally recommended ELDI sage and should be used in the following indications:

- Tumors
- Painful skin areas
- Metastases
- Hepatic impairment and liver support
- Kidney problems
- Bladder disorders
- Intestinal cramps
- Lung disorders

- Bone disorders of all kinds

ELDI Oil Enema

Enemas are used in the Oil-Protein Diet exclusively for the energy intake and not for the purification of the intestine. Dr Budwig used to give ELDI oil or Flax oil enema to her serious patients. Budwig used to get immediate and miraculous results with the most seriously ill patients. Flax seed Oil enema also give similar results.

I recommend you to make the first enemas only with 100ml and then increase over several days to 250ml. Some patients have enemas with 500ml oil and positively reported on it. 500ml are however the absolute exception and mostly not necessary. Usually 250ml suffice.

Incidentally, smaller amounts are also easily introduced with an enema syringe instead of with an enema bucket. Enema syringes are available in sizes up to 350ml and are easy to handle.

Standard plan for ELDI oil R: Day 1 = 100ml, day 2 = 100ml, day 3 = 150ml, day 4 = 150ml, day 5 = 200ml, day 6 = 200ml and day 7 = 250ml.

From the seventh day, one remains at 250ml, and so long until the patient is significantly better. Then you can go back to 100ml - 150ml, always together with 1-2 daily whole body rubbings. (Oil Protein Diet by Lothar Hirneise)

Ingredients

- Enema pot
- Watch
- A bowl to collect oil when you are getting rid of bubbles.
- Towel and tissue
- RO filtered water
- ELDI oil or Flax oil
- Towel or Drip Stand

Procedure

Prepare a place near the toilet, so that if you can't hold the enema, you will be making a quick dash and the shorter distance is better.

Cleansing Enema with Plain water

First of all you should take a plain water enema. Purpose of this enema is cleaning of intestines. It is not a retention enema and is evacuated immediately. For this you may use 500-1000ml (2-4 cups) RO filtered water. As soon as the whole water is inside the rectum, go and sit on the commode and release the water slowly.

Take the oil enema immediately after the water enema

- Use advised (above) amount of ELDI or Flax oil. The oil should be at body temperature. The best test is to dip your little finger into the oil.
- Fill the oil into the enema pot. It takes at least 5 minutes for the bubbles to get out of the tube.
- The enema pot should be hanged on a drip stand about 2-3 feet above your body.
- You need to lubricate the nozzle and anus with Flax oil. When all is ready, lie on your right side in the fetal position. Insert the nozzle into the rectum slowly and carefully with your left hand, and un-pinch the tube.
- If you feel little uncomfortable when the oil is going in, pinch the tube, wait till the feeling passes away, then continue again.
- The oil is much more viscous and moves more slowly. You might need to hold the pot a bit higher to get it to run a bit quicker.
- Once the oil is in, wait and hold it for about 12 minutes. After that slowly turn yourself to left side and hold oil for

another 12 minutes. You may listen to music while taking enema.

- When done, it is best to sit on the commode for about 15 minutes with something to read (Skelton).

Coffee Enema

Dr. Max Gerson introduced coffee enema back in the 1930s. In this enema about 500ml of coffee is pushed into rectum, this amount only reaches up to sigmoid colon. There is no loss of minerals and electrolytes in Coffee Enema because their absorption occurs well before sigmoid colon. Coffee enema is even safe for those who are allergic to coffee because it is not absorbed into the systemic circulation. You may take this enema once or twice. It has the following benefits:

- **Powerful and Natural Pain Reliever**
- **Cleansing** - Coffee also acts as an astringent in the large intestine, helps cleanse the colon walls.
- **Toxin Elimination** - The major benefit of the coffee enema is elimination of toxins through the liver. Caffeine, theophylline and theobromine dilate the blood vessels and bile ducts, stimulate the liver to discharge more bile and boost the detoxifying process into high gear and heal inflammation. Indeed, endoscopic studies confirm they increase bile output.
- **Stimulates Liver** - Kahweol and cafestol palmitate found in coffee promote the activity of a key enzyme system called glutathione S-Transferase. This is an important mechanism in the detoxification of carcinogens, as the enzyme group is responsible for neutralizing free radicals.

Coffee enema stimulates the activity of this system by 600- 700%.

Coffee Enema Procedure

- This enema is retained for 12-14 minutes, during this time blood circulates in liver three times and blood is purified. Coffee enema can be given several times a day, few patients take up to seven times a day. Normally if pain is not relieved it may be taken more than one time. You should relax while taking enema; you may listen to music or read newspaper while relaxing. The best time for coffee enema is either early morning after you passed motion or during the day time.
- Grind organic coffee beans. Put approx. 750ml of filtered water in a steal pan and bring it to boil. Add 2-5 heaped Tbsp coffee powder, 3 Tbsp is ideal. It is roughly 20-25grams. Let it continue to simmer for ten minutes or more and then turn off the burner. Allow it to cool down to a very comfortable, tepid temperature. Test it with your finger. It should be the same temperature as your body's temperature. Filter the coffee with fine mesh steal sieve into a jug. This is approximately 500ml.
- Pour 2 cups (500ml) of coffee into the enema pot. Be sure the plastic hose is clamped tightly. Now open the clamp and grasp, but do not close the clamp on the hose. Place the enema tip in the sink. Hold up the enema bag above the tip until the coffee begins to flow out. As soon as it starts flowing, quickly close the clamp. This expels any air in the tube.
- Lubricate the enema tip with a small amount of coconut oil or KY jelly. Create a comfortable and relaxing atmosphere. After a few days you will thoroughly enjoy this ritual.
- Light a candle, play some light music and most importantly, make sure you are comfortable and warm.

We recommend placing a pillow with a washable cover under your head and lying down on an old towel.

- The position preferred is lying on your back. With the clamp closed hang the pot about 3 feet above your belly. We like to hang the enema pot on a drip stand.
- Insert the tip gently into anus and open the clamp slowly. You should relax and breathe. The coffee may take a few seconds to begin flowing. If you develop a cramp, close the hose clamp, turn from side to side and take a few deep breaths. The cramp will usually pass quickly. Usually nothing happens.
- When all the liquid is inside, close the clamp and remove it slowly. Retain the enema for 12- 14 minutes. You may remain lying on the floor.
- After 14 minutes or so, go to the toilet and empty your gut. Take your time. Wash the enema pot and tube thoroughly with soap and water.
- Take more potassium in the form of fruits and vegetable juices if you take coffee enema regularly (S.A.Wilsons.com).

Epsom bath

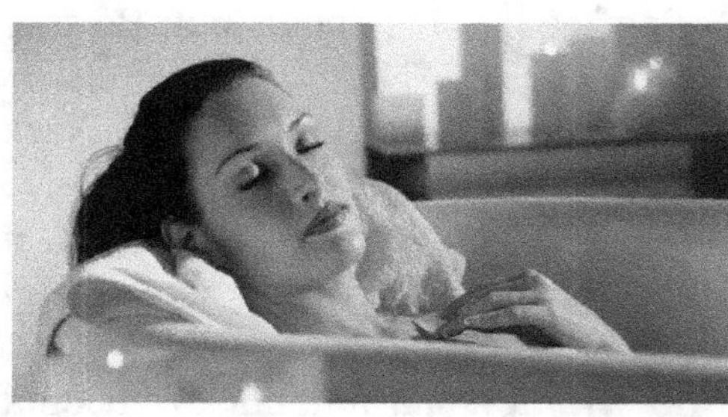

Detoxification of your body through bathing is an ancient remedy that anyone can perform in the comfort of your own home. Your skin is known as the third kidney, and toxins are excreted through sweating. An Epsom salt bath is thought to assist your body in eliminating toxins as well as absorbing the magnesium and nutrients that are in the water. Soaking in Epsom salt actually helps replenish the body's magnesium levels, combating hypertension. The sulfate flushes toxins and helps form proteins in brain tissue and joints. Most of all, it will leave you relaxed, refreshed and awakened. Take it once a week or as advised.

Prepare your bath

- It is a 40 minutes ritual. The first 20 minutes are said to help your body remove the toxins, while the second 20 minutes are for absorbing the minerals from the water
- Fill your tub with comfortably hot water. Use a chlorine filter if possible.
- Add Epsom salt (Magnesium sulfate). For people 50 Kg and up, add 2 cups or more to a standard bath tub.
- Then add 2 cups or more of soda bicarb. It is known for its cleansing ability and even has anti-fungal properties. It also leaves skin very soft.
- Add 2-3 Tbsp ground ginger. While this step is optional, ginger can increase your heat levels, helping to sweat out more toxins. However, since it is heating the body, it may cause your skin to turn slightly red for a few minutes, so be careful with the amount you add. Depending on the capacity of your tub, anywhere from 1 Tbsp to 1/3 cup can be added (Herneise).
- Add aromatherapy oils. Again optional, but there are many oils that will make the bath an even more pleasant and relaxing experience (such as lavender), as well as those that will assist in the detoxification process (tea tree or eucalyptus oil). Around 20 drops is sufficient for a standard bath.
- Swish all of the ingredients around in the tub, and then slip into the tub. You should start sweating within the first few minutes. If you feel too hot, start adding cold water into the tub until you cool off.
- Get out of the tub slowly and carefully. Your body has been working hard and you may get lightheaded or feel weak and drained. On top of that, the salts make your tub slippery, so stand with care.

- Drink plenty of water and relax in bed for a few minutes

Soda bicarb bath

Lothar Hirneise has given lot of importance to Soda bicarb bath. It is thought to assist you in eliminating toxins as well as making your body alkaline so your tumor cells may suffocate. Patient may take it once or even twice a day. Just add 2 cups of soda bicarb in your bath tub filled with warm water and relax in it for 30-40 minutes (Hirneise, 2005).

Sun Therapy

Getting an adequate amount of sunshine is a critical part of Budwig protocol. Once the body has acquired the right oil-protein balance with the Cottage Cheeseand Flax oil, the body develops better capacity to absorb the healing photons from the sun. Remember that for healing of cancer high energy photons from the sun are very important. The sunshine is important to maintain adequate vitamin-D levels in our body. Vitamin-D is a powerful antioxidant that has been linked to preventing many diseases including cancer.

Dr. Budwig's focus was on the importance of photons from the sunbeams and their interaction with vital essential fats (linoleic and linolenic acid) in our body. It is the interaction of photons from the sun and the electrons in proper food that provide the synergistic effect on healing our body. Eating the electron rich Flax oil/Cottage Cheese mixture, must be connected with adequate exposure to sunlight.

There is nothing else on earth with a higher concentration of photons of the sun's energy than man. This concentration of the sun's energy is very much energetic point for humans, with their wave eminently suitable lengths - is improved when we eat electron rich essential oils, which in turn absorbs the photons in the form of electro-magnetic waves of sunbeams.

When you eat the FO/CC mixture, your body becomes a better antenna for the photons from the sunbeam. Your body develops a better ability to absorb the energy from the sun and Transfer it to your cells to perform their vital functions. You become energized at a deep level, and when this happens cancer is healed itself.

It is red light that penetrates deeper in the tissues. In 1968 Dr. Budwig used 695 nm ruby (red) lasers light with success to radiate healthy surrounding cancer tissues in cancer patients.

How long should you take this protocol?

If all is well patient feels better and tumor start to shrink within a 3 or 4 months, if he follows treatment religiously and honestly. He may be cured in one or two years. **It is recommended that the Budwig protocol and full diet is followed for at least five years.** Even after that he should maintain healthy eating and life style.

Dr. Budwig has clearly mentioned that if you do not get the desired success, do not blame the protocol, rather try to find out your mistakes and correct them. The threshold between winning and losing is very small, and even a minor mistake can unbalance the complete healing process.

Linomel

Linomel is an invention by Dr Budwig. Freshly crushed Flax seed is mixed with honey and milk powder so that the crushed Flax seed is more stable. There is no doubt that freshly crushed Flax seed is more valuable, but also has the disadvantage that you do it yourself and clean the grinder afterwards. That is why Linomel still has an existence right. Do not buy crushed Flax seed in the shop as the chance that these contain Trans fatty acids is 100%.

Is there an alternative to Linomel?

- Freshly crushed Flax seed is an alternative. This must be eaten immediately after the meal, otherwise it will oxidize.
- Make your own Linomel. Mix 6 tablespoons freshly crushed Flax seed with a tablespoon of honey. Small tip: Grind the Flax seed, e.g. in a coffee grinder, and set the grinder to coarse. So it mixes better with the honey.

(Oil Protein Diet by Lothar Hieneise)

Daylight

Dr Budwig focused upon the importance of daylight to our health. It is not enough to absorb electrons only through food, but it is important that we feed ourselves so that our cells are able to absorb and process the light coming from the sun. The more sickly someone is, the sooner he is "in the house", which can be a catastrophic mistake. Especially when people are already in a very late stage of the illness, they are often not able to eat enough and good advice is then very difficult. In such cases, Dr Budwig advises to concentrate on the following three points:

- ELDI oils as whole body rubbings and if possible as enemas
- Only freshly squeezed juices and distributed as food throughout the day if possible the breakfast muesli in different variants
- Stay outside as much as possible

You will experience me to explain what to do next. I have been able to see in my life how Dr Budwig's theoretical considerations work when put to practice, if indeed, if they are consistently carried out. If you could experience such a case yourself, and how quickly it can be better for a seriously ill person, you can see Dr Budwig's words in a very different light.

But other great researchers had also dealt with the subject of light long before Dr Budwig. For example, the anthroposophist Rudolf Steiner wrote, about 50 years earlier that there is a fundamental being of our material existence of the earth, of which all materiality has come only through condensation. Every matter on earth is condensed light! There is nothing in material existence, which is something else than condensed light in some form. Wherever you go and feel matter, you have condensed light everywhere. Compressed light. Matter is light by its very nature. In as much as a man is a material being, he is woven of light. Rudolf Steiner and Dr Budwig have pointed out in their writings over and over again the importance of light and that we humans are now heliotropes, which need light and use light. But I have nowhere else than with Dr Budwig so clearly and understandably read, WHY this is and above all, how the charging of the life battery works and / or what importance mainly the linolenic acid or electron clouds play. Because it is so important, I would like to repeat here again: The sicklier someone is, the more he should be in the open." (Oil-Protein Diet by Lothar Hirneise)

Disclaimer

This book is not intended to replace the advice and/or care of a qualified health care professional. Please do not try to self diagnose or self treat any disease. Seek professional help and consult your physician before making any dietary changes.

This book is not intended to provide medical advice and is sold with the understanding that the publisher and the author have neither liability nor responsibility to any person or entity with respect to loss, damage or injury caused or alleged to be caused directly or indirectly by the information contained in this book or the use of any products mentioned. Readers should not use any of the product discussed in this book without the advice of a medical profession.

The Food and Drug Administration has not approved the use of any of the natural treatments discussed in this book. This book, and the information contained herein, has not been approved by the Food and the Drug Administration.

Cancer - Cause and Cure
Based on Quantum Physics developed by Dr. Johanna Budwig

http://www.amazon.com/Cancer-Quantum-Physics-developed-Johanna-ebook/dp/B00P3Y7BYG

Book Description

***** A must have book for every cancer patient *****

This book provides an introduction of Dr. Budwig's cancer research and treatment. Johanna

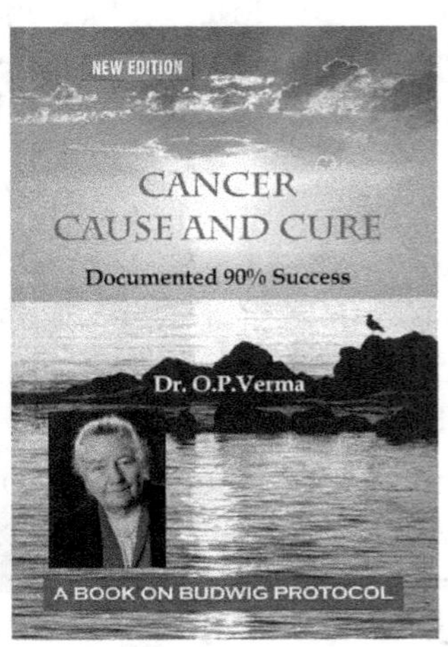

Budwig (1908-2003) was nominated for the Nobel Prize seven times. She was one of Germany's leading scientists of the 20th Century, a biochemist and cancer specialist with a special interest in essential fats.

Otto Warburg proved that prime cause of cancer oxygen-deficiency in the cells. In absence of oxygen cells ferment glucose to produce energy, lactic acid is formed as a byproduct of fermentation. He postulated that sulfur containing protein and some unknown fat is required to attract oxygen in the cell.

In 1951 Dr. Budwig developed Paper Chromatography to identify fats. With this technique she proved that electron rich highly unsaturated Linoleic and Linolenic fatty acids were the undiscovered mysterious decisive fats in respiratory enzyme function that Otto Warburg had been unable to find. She studied the electromagnetic function of pi-electrons of the linolenic acid in the membranes of the microstructure of protoplasm, for all nerve function, secretions, mitosis, as well as cell break-down. This immediately caused lot of excitement in the scientific community. New doors could open in Cancer research. Hydrogenated fats, including all Trans fatty acids were proved as respiratory poisons.

Then Budwig decided to have human trials and gave flaxseed oil and quark to cancer patients. After three months, the patients began to improve in health and strength, the yellow green substance in their blood began to disappear, tumors gradually receded and at the same time the nutrients began to rise. This way Dr. Budwig had found a cure for cancer. It was a great victory and first milestone in the battle against cancer. Her treatment protocol is based on the consumption of flax seed oil with low fat cottage cheese, raw organic diet, mild exercise, and the healing powers of the sun. She treated approx. 2500 cancer patients during a 50 year period with this protocol till her death with over 90% documented success.

She was nominated 7 times for Nobel Prize but with a condition that she will use chemotherapy and radiotherapy with her protocol. They did not want to collapse the 200 billion dollar business over night. She always refused to support the damaging chemo and radio for the sake of humanity.

The book also, describes about rare and miraculous herbs used in the treatment of Cancer like Turmeric, Black seed, Ginger, Mistle Toe, Aloe vera, Echinecea, Lobelia, Essiac Tea, Pau d'arco Tea, Dandelion, Milk Thistle.

~~**~~

Cancer Cure Is Found: Letrile is the answer

https://www.amazon.com/Cancer-Cure-Found-Laetrile-
answer/dp/1797710206/

CANCER CURE IS FOUND

During 1950, a biochemist Dr. Ernest T. Krebs Jr., isolated a new vitamin from bitter apricot kernel that he called 'B-17' or 'Laetrile'. He conducted further lab animal and culture experiments to conclude that laetrile would be effective in the treatment of cancer. He proposed that cancer was caused by a deficiency of Vitamin B 17 (Laetrile, Amygdaline). Laetrile is a concentrated and purified form of vitamin B17. After a lot of research, he had finally developed a specific protocol to treat cancer. Laetrile Therapy combines Laetrile with nutritional supplements and a healthy diet to create a potent treatment that fights cancer cells while helping to strengthen the body's immune system.

Vitamin B-17, which is present in several different foods, consists of a locked substance which comprises two units' glucose, one unit benzaldehyde and one unit cyanide. When B17 comes in contact with a cancer cell it is unlocked by a hormone found only in the cancer cell, and becomes a lethal chemical bomb which destroys the cancer cell. Healthy cells do not cause breakdown of B17. Cancer is unknown to people living in areas with food products rich in B-17, and the population lives to a remarkably high age. Apparently nature has provided us with an ingenious defense against cancer, and it is an

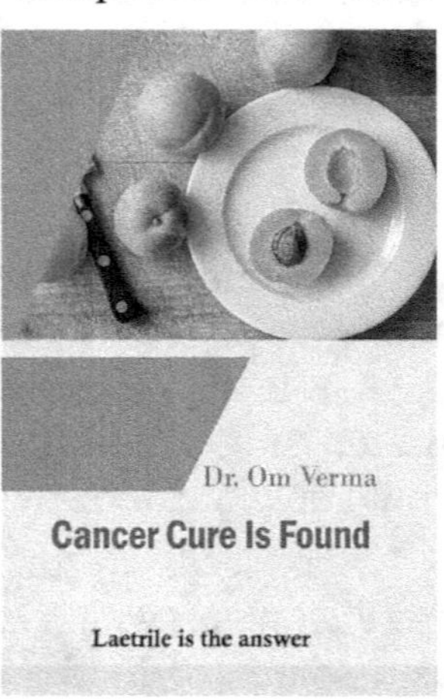

ordinary nutrient in our food. These are, amongst others nuts, seeds, vegetables, and in particular apricot kernels.

At present, patients listen or read a lot about Laetrile treatment, but usually they don't get precise and to the point information about what are the exact components of this protocol, where to get Laetrile injections and supplements, what to take, what not to take, what are the doses, how long to take the treatment, what diet they have to follow, etc. In this book, I have explained the protocol in detail proposed by Dr. Krebs. I have given every minute detail about Laetrile, other nutritional supplements and diet in this book. After reading this book patients can buy Laetrile injections, tablets and other nutritional supplements from the reliable sources (given in the book) and conduct the treatment under the supervision of their family doctor. Dr. Philip E. Binzel was personally trained by Dr. Ernest T. Kreb Jr. about everything of this treatment. Dr. Binzel had been using Laetrile therapy in the treatment of cancer patients since the mid 1970s. His record of success was astounding. Testimonies of his patients are also included in this book.

Available on Amazon.in
Awesome Flax: A Book by Flax Guru
Flax seed- Miraculous Anti-ageing Divine Food

What is Flax seed and how can it benefit me? I was faced with this question when I started hearing about Flax seed not long ago. It became a 'buzz word' in society and seems to be making great role in increased health for many. I wanted to join that wagon of wellness and so I researched until I felt satisfied that it could help me, too. Here are my findings.

Flax seeds are the hard, tiny seeds of Linum usitatissimum, the Flax plant, which has been widely used for thousands of years as a source of food and clothing. Flax seeds have become very popular recently, because they are a richest source of the Omega

3 essential fatty acid; also known as Alpha Linolenic Acid (ALA) and lignans. People in the new millennium may see Flax seed as an important new FOOD SUPER STAR. In fact, there's nobody who won't benefit by adding Flax seed to his or her diet. Even Gandhi wrote: "Wherever Flax seed becomes a regular food item among the people, there will be better health."

Flax seed contains 30-40% oil (including 36-50% alpha linolenic acid, 23-24% linoleic acid- Omega-6 fatty acids and oleic acids), mucilage (6%), protein (25%), Vitamin B group, lecithin, selenium, calcium, folate, magnesium, zinc, iron, carotene, sulfur, potassium, phosphorous, manganese, silicon, copper, nickel, molybdenum, chromium, and cobalt, vitamins A and E and all essential amino acids.

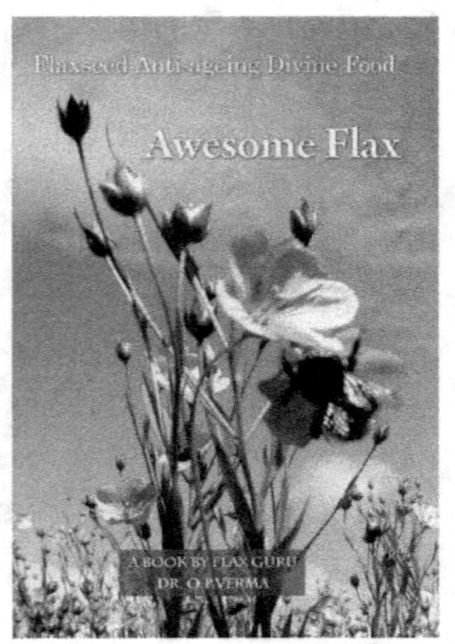

Other fatty acids, omega-6's, is abundant in vegetable oils such as corn, soybean, safflower, and sunflower oils as well as in the many processed foods made from these oils. Omega-6 fatty acids have stimulating, irritating and inflammatory effect while omega-3 fatty acids have calming and soothing effect on our body. Our bodies function best when our diets contain a well-balanced ratio of these fatty acids, meaning 1:1 to 4:1 of omega-6 and omega-3. But we typically eat 10 to 30 times more omega-6's than omega-3's, which is a prescription for trouble. This imbalance puts us at greater risk for a number of serious illnesses, including heart disease, cancer, stroke, and arthritis. As the most abundant plant source of omega-3 fatty acids, Flax seed helps restore balance and lets omega-3's do what they're best at: balancing the immune system, decreasing inflammation, and lowering some of the risk factors for heart disease.

One way that Omega 3 essential fatty acid known as Alpha Linolenic Acid ALA helps the heart is by decreasing the ability of platelets to clump together. Flax seed helps to lower high blood pressure, clears clogged coronaries, lowers high blood cholesterol, bad LDL cholesterol and triglyceride levels and raises good HDL cholesterol. It can relieve the symptoms of Diabetes Mellitus. It lowers blood sugar level. Flax seed help fight obesity. Adding Flax seed to foods creates a feeling of satiation. Furthermore, Flax seed stokes the metabolic processes in our cells. Much like a furnace, once stoked, the cells generate more heat and burn calories.

Flax seeds are the most abundant source of lignans. Lignans are plant-based compounds that can block estrogen activity in cells, reducing the risk of Breast, Uterus, Colon and Prostate cancers. According to the US Department of Agriculture, Flax seed contains 27 identifiable cancer preventative compounds. Lignans in Flax seeds are 200 to 800 times more than any other lignan source. Lignans are phytoestrogens, meaning that they are similar to but weaker than the estrogen that a woman's body produces naturally. Therefore, they may also help alleviate menopausal discomforts such as hot flashes and vaginal dryness. They are also antibacterial, antifungal, and antiviral.

Because they are high in dietary fiber, ground Flax seeds can help ease the passage of stools and thus relieve constipation, hemorrhoids and diverticular disease. Taken for inflammatory bowel disease, Flax seed can help to calm inflammation and repair any intestinal tract damage.

Multiple Myeloma New Horizon

With Orthodox and Alternative Treatments

https://www.amazon.com/Multiple-Myeloma-New-Horizon-Alternative/dp/1797876015/

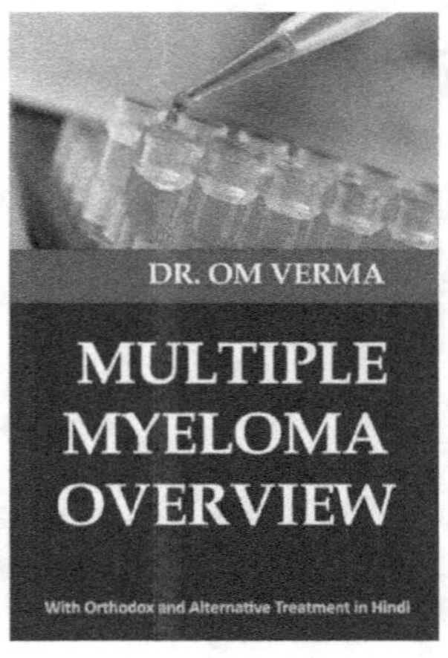

I have written this book so that the patients suffering from multiple myeloma can understand the disease in detail and choose a suitable treatment for them. This book provides detailed information about the clinical symptoms, complications, diagnosis, staging and treatments. In the last 15 years there has been considerable research and progress in the field of clinical studies, etiology, pathology, diagnosis and treatment of multiple myeloma. Even if we do not have the cure of this disease, but still it is one of the highly treatable disease today. Today we have new and effective medicines, which work in a much better way. There are new treatments for bone lesions and fractures. There are new resources for the treatment of its complications. Not long ago, life of a Myeloma patient was miserable, confined to a wheelchair and he barely survived 2-3 years. At present time, Multiple Myeloma patients are surviving 10 years or more and are living comfortable life. The lifestyle of the patient is getting happier and convenient.

In this book, I have written in detail about Orthodox and Alternative Treatment (Budwig Protocol, which is the best alternative treatment and gives authentic success). Patient can carefully select the right treatment for him. This book has up to date information.